# Food Truths,
# Food Lies

# Food Truths, Food Lies

## Take Control of Your Diet, Your Weight, and Your Health

Eric A. Marcotte, M.D.

# MFW Press, USA

Dedicated to my patients –
past, present, and future

# Table of Contents

# Introduction

I've never had a day as a doctor when I haven't been asked for help with someone's weight in one way or another. Sometimes it's a direct request, even the reason I'm seeing the person. "Doc, I can't lose." "Doc, help me." "Give me something to help me lose."

Other times it's more roundabout, or even starts with me. "Mr. Jones, your sugar is really climbing and you're going to be diabetic soon if we can't find a way to bring your weight down."

No matter who starts it, the subject seems to make people despair. Who really has had long term success with their weight? Some lucky folks never seem to struggle with it at all. This book isn't for them. I doubt they'd even pick it up.

Some people have had great success losing weight and keeping it off, even large amounts, like Subway Jared. I have to say, I've seen this pretty rarely. One, maybe two people in a hundred can permanently lose more than ten or fifteen pounds without artificial help.

There are a growing number of people who have lost weight over the long-term using some powerful help, usually stomach-changing major surgery that they are willing to risk their lives on. For those that are truly dying from their weight, this may seem their only real option and thousands more choose it every year.

As a doctor, I'm by no means against "bariatric surgery," this stomach closing, intestine re-routing method of helping desperate people lose the weight that is killing them. I've referred dozens of people to the expert surgeons in my area for this life-changing procedure. I've also seen nearly every complication the surgery can cause. Patients can lose half their body weight or more but often become permanently sick in the process, unable to ever properly digest again.

This type of surgery is a last resort for people who feel they have reached the end of their options and are willing to gamble to get their lives back. This book probably isn't for them either. There are people who truly cannot control their eating, who have food addictions complicated by terrible genes and lifelong wrong attitudes about food. Many of these folks need to have their entire system changed by surgery. I do not discourage those that truly need surgery from pursuing it, though I try to be careful and educate them about the risks they are taking.

So this book isn't for the naturally lean, the rare permanent weight loss success story or those dying from their obesity that need surgery to survive. Who is it for? I am writing to the thousands of other patients I've known and the many millions of other regular people who struggle with their weight and health.  Statistics say that there are over 100 million people who fit this last category in the US alone.

If I'm talking to one of them right now, I think you may be in the right place, reading the right book.  I want to get into food in a way I've never seen another author do it.  I want to help teach people to know their food.  I want choosing the right foods to be as natural as choosing the right outfit.  If I had my way, this teaching would be done and learned by the time a kid was about a third grader. Everyone would know their food like they know their alphabet and multiplication tables.

Nutrition education, deeply known and acted on, would solve many of our problems with weight (and maybe bankrupt McDonald's and a few other deserving companies along the way.)

Unfortunately, if you're old enough to drive to the bookstore and browse this introduction, you're probably past the point where it's easy to learn new habits – what we often call "adulthood."  Now, don't get me wrong.  There are lots of good things about being an adult besides having a driver's license and a credit card, and adults are absolutely capable of learning new habits.

It's just not easy.  It's not.  Simply put, adults learn facts much more easily than children but learn behaviors much less easily than when they were children.  That makes a book like this so important.  The facts need to be learn-able and the reasons to learn them plain and the motivation to change obvious.

I've talked to thousands of folks that want to lose weight and learned some things from them and about them along the way.

First, change only happens when someone wants to change. Whether it's quitting cigarettes or Burger King or excess TV, "it's a free country" as I remind my patients and myself every day.  I have never and will never make someone lose weight and probably can't even make them want to lose weight.  The best I can do is coax, teach, encourage, inform, and support.

That's the best this book can do too.  If there is no "want to" in you right now, please look elsewhere for it.  These pages will not _make_ you do anything.  What I hope I can do for you and with you is to open your eyes to habits, wrong information, and bad thinking about our bodies and the food we need to keep them in good working order.

Earlier, I mentioned that my wish was to teach these things early in childhood, making life much easier for adults with good habits and good knowledge.  The problem isn't really that no one learns about food as a child.  Instead of simply no teaching on food and nutrition for kids, there actually is lots of <u>bad</u> teaching going on. It starts before we even learn to talk and is pretty well formed before we reach puberty.

Our parents are our first teachers about food and everything else. Some of the things you know about food and nutrition was learned before you could crawl. Eating made you happy and you eating made your parents happy. Eating was a game and a fun one for most babies and toddlers. What, when, and why we eat gets programmed in our high chair, all while smearing and throwing baby food everywhere.

Playmates, teachers and television all have a lot of power over what kids learn too. All of this education in nutrition comes way before we learn algebra and is ingrained much deeper than any multiplication table ever could be.

That makes our job with this book tougher but also more important. Tougher because many of the things I want to teach you may at first seem wrong and you may not even know why. The <u>why</u> could be because you learned it when you were still chewing on your blocks instead of stacking them. It's hard to fight against stuff we learned so early, but we have to. We have to if we want to be different and if we want our children and their children to have it easier than we have. If you learned this stuff with a bib on, so are your children. If you know better, they can know better and your grandchildren might not even have to unlearn the wrong stuff.

But it has to start somewhere and I dare you to start it now. Learn, change, make the first step to a new way of thinking, eating, and weighing start now. Read on.

Many of our favorite foods, often the ones we learned to eat as kids, are so full of calories that a reasonable serving size has a completely unreasonable number of calories. This gives us a very difficult problem. The foods I like in the amounts I want have so many calories I'll need to buy bigger pants every year or so. Sound familiar?

This is the heart of why I have had so many conversations with frustrated patients over their weight. This is exactly why I'm writing this book. This is the rub that may make some of you want to put down this book in despair – don't! You've got to hang in there with me and learn to make new choices or you will never succeed in your goal of changing your weight. It's that simple.

> **Permanent change in your weight absolutely requires change in your eating and your thinking about your eating.**

Read that sentence again if you need to. The rest of this book won't help at all if we get stuck here. Some of you are getting uncomfortable right about now. Maybe there's a little grumbling going on.  "I spent $20 to hear that I have to change?  I know that!  How?"

Like I said, hang in there.  The **how** will take us chapters to completely understand.  Right now, I want us to all agree that our food choices and weights aren't what they should be and that we want to be different.  If that's still true for you, read on.  If not, hopefully the bookstore won't notice your highlighting – try to get your $20 back.

# Truth and Lies

You're being lied to. It happens every day, all day long. The problem is, the lies come so fast and thick and have been flying for so long that they don't seem like lies anymore. We sure don't call them lies. We have lots of nicer names for this stuff, like *advertising* or *menus* or *magazines*.

When a child lies to his teacher and then calls it a fib or a story or an excuse, the teacher doesn't smile and pat him on the head. If the teacher knows it's a lie, I'd bet the kid gets called to the principal's office and mom may get a call too.

So why don't we call the CEO of Kraft or McDonald's when we find them lying to us? I think it's because we usually don't even know we're being lied to. Nearly everything we read, hear, or see goes along with the lies so much that they just seem part of everyday normal life.

I want to look at some of these lies and show you that they are lies and talk about what's really true instead. Why companies or media or anyone else lies about food and nutrition is just my opinion. That they are lying is easy to prove with some simple detective work. I want you to learn to do your own detective work and learn to see through the lies.

The lies come in many forms, from the bold lie, like a full-of-sugar kid's cereal claiming to be healthy to the subtle lie, like the extra-value sized portions at many restaurants. The lies are so common that **I think you are safe to assume that every food package, advertisement, or menu is lying to you.** From what I can see, at least 99% of them are and I'll just personally apologize to the two or three ethical companies out there when I find them. The rest? Liars.

If you stick with me over the next several chapters, I'll show you the lies and the methods for lying that these companies use. Here and there I'll even get into some theories about why they are lying, but for now, just follow the money and you'll have a general idea why we're being lied to. It works, that's why. These lies sell more food to more people than corporate honesty and openness would, so, surprise, here come the lies.

I think that if the average shopper knew, really knew what he or she was buying and actually eating, we would be a much thinner and healthier nation and the food companies would offer much leaner, healthier foods. Unfortunately, nearly every shopper at your local store is clueless about the calories in their food and just wants what tastes good or is convenient or has a pretty package in the amount that makes them feel good and full. So, this is exactly what the food companies put on the shelves.

And the result of that shopper ignorance and corporate greed?  Millions of overweight, unhealthy, tired, and frustrated people.  My secret hope is that this book can help start a change in enough people to pressure the food companies to label more honestly and sell more responsibly.

Companies are run to make money.  Any company that isn't making money is headed for bankruptcy.  So it shouldn't come as a surprise that companies do whatever makes them the most money.  Expecting ethical decisions by a corporation is just wishful thinking and I don't think we can change that.  What can be changed are the attitudes and appetites and education of the people who buy those companies' products.  If you and I, the average shoppers and restaurant-goers, had some basic knowledge about food and nutrition, the companies selling their food would be forced to stop telling certain lies, because those lies wouldn't work.

That is exactly what I want for us, what I want for my patients and my readers and maybe for our society as a whole.  I want us to learn to look a menu or ingredient label in the eye and make the healthy choice.  If enough of us do this often enough maybe we can change those companies.

If you and me and every other shopper knew that "Trans-fat FREE!" is hogwash and that portraying juice as healthy should make an advertiser's nose grow, these lies would disappear and we would have healthier, reasonably portioned and more honestly labeled food to buy at the store or restaurant. These are a few of the many things we have to talk about in the following pages.

You'll learn to see the lie behind "Now fat free!" and "100% wheat goodness" and "Part of a healthy breakfast" and the 20 ounce soda pop. By the time you get through this little book, I want you to be picking out new food lies - they're everywhere - and writing to tell me about the worst or funniest ones.

# The First Truth

The greatest teacher said "The truth will set you free," so we'll start with some simple truths first. I hope this will make it easier to see the lies when we start looking for them.

The **First Truth** we need to know is that **calories count**. Food companies and diet companies both would rather you didn't know this truth. In the simplest terms the human body is a machine. To be sure, it is an amazing and unbelievably complicated machine. But if we think of it as a machine then we can get to the simple but incredibly important truth that calories really do count. I often tell my patients that even one extra calorie a day will lead to weight gain and even one calorie too few a day will lead to weight loss. Now since there are 3,500 or so calories to a pound, a one calorie difference per day will take a long time to change your weight. But if you do the math, as little as 10 calories a day can really start to add up. One after-dinner mint usually has around 10 calories (though some have a lot more.) You can calculate that one mint a day for a year will equal a pound. A mint is a pound? Yup, you read right. Ten calories is "nothing" - one mint, one crouton, a stick of gum – yet it can add up that fast.

What if this were 100 calories extra a day instead of a measly ten? 100 calories a day can make nearly a pound a month difference and 500 calories a day will make a pound a week difference. All of this is simple but powerful math and can't be fooled by any fancy diet plan.

A person that is serious about weight loss and who wants to keep the weight off rather than have it come right back must learn how many calories their food has. Every diet that has ever worked for anyone has worked because that person has eaten fewer calories than their body needed on a regular basis. No matter what method you use, if your body demands more calories than it takes in, it will have to go to its savings account (fat supply) and make a withdrawal. When you do this to your checkbook that is a bad thing and we call it bouncing a check. When you do this to your waist line we usually think it's a good thing and call it losing weight.

Let's go back to our simple math for a minute. Because I have learned to pay attention to my food I know even without looking that a can of Coke has 150 calories in it. I know that a Big Mac has over 500 calories and that a Snickers bar has almost 300. I guess you can tell the things I used to eat regularly before I started learning about calories, huh? Now when I think of a can of Coke I automatically multiply it for the year and realize that is 16 pounds. A Big Mac? How about 52 pounds?

Before I turn everyone into an anorexic, remember that these are round estimates and that our bodies are not perfectly efficient when we burn food as energy. What I want my patients and you to know is how absolutely essential it is to be aware of what you're putting in your mouth and what affect that will have on your weight.

These calorie estimates become more accurate and even more important as we consider the Second Truth.

# The Second Truth

The First Truth will make snack food companies and fast food restaurants mad at me.  The Second Truth will tick off my gym manager.

The **Second Truth** is that **you can't exercise your way to weight loss**.  Very few people can "burn off" enough calories to be able to lose weight without changing their eating habits.  Once again, grade school math can help us out here.  Most gyms have treadmills that will tell you how many calories you've burned using your age, sex, weight and effort to calculate.  As a rough estimate, a 200 pound man that's 40 years old can burn 10 calories a minute with a fast walk or slow jog.  The speed most people walk, it takes almost twice as long.  It will take even longer to burn those 10 calories if you're older, weigh less than 200 pounds or are a woman because of how body chemistry works.

If we use our math and new knowledge of Coke (150 calories per can) we can estimate that most people take 20-30 minutes of walking to burn off one can of Coke.  Seems pretty unfair, doesn't it?  When I'm thirsty I can down a can of Coke in a minute or two.  To think that one minute of refreshment will take a half hour of walking to burn off is a little overwhelming, but that is the honest truth.

Let's look at how long it will take to burn off a pound of fat. A pound of fat is about 3,500 calories. If that fast-walking man wants to burn a pound of fat at the gym, he better pack a lunch (which then puts him even further behind!) It will take him over 10 hours of fast, sweaty walking to lose one pound!

Exercise is great for your heart, gives you energy and takes away stress, and is essential to weight maintenance, but really won't cut it for weight loss, at least not alone.

# The Third Truth

Our First Truth is that calories count.  The Second Truth comes from the first and shows how much easier it is to keep calories away (by not eating them in the first place) than it is to burn them off once they move in around our waists.

The Third Truth is comes from the first two.  (Surprised?  I told you calories matter!)

This Third Truth will make everyone else mad at me who isn't already.  The First Truth made the food and restaurant companies mad, the Second Truth made the gyms and exercise machine companies mad.  This one will probably make you mad, but since it's true, don't you want to hear it anyway?

The **Third Truth** is that **the first two truths matter more than who you are.**  What I mean is that what you eat and how fast you try to burn it off are more important than your genes, your metabolism, and your thyroid put together.  See?  I told you I'd make you mad.

The conversations I have with my patients always end up butting heads with this truth and I do a lot of blood tests to help prove to people that this truth is true.  It goes something like this:

Dr. Marcotte, my mom's best friend's aunt found out she had thyroid trouble that her doctor never looked for. He just told her she was fat and needed to eat less for years and years. I looked on the Internet and I have all the symptoms and I think that's why I can never lose weight.

Now, I'm a reasonable guy, and I sure don't want to mess up like that poor lady's bad doctor, so I agree to test Ms. Smith. I always try to prepare her for the Third Truth, though. I usually plan another appointment a few weeks later, so we can weigh her again and look at her thyroid tests and anything else her symptoms suggest might be out of whack. I also gently warn her that I think the tests will all be normal and that we'll have to look elsewhere for a way to lose weight.

The problem is the Third Truth is true. Even if there is a thyroid problem (and a lot of people do have thyroid trouble, don't misunderstand me) I have never found the thyroid to be responsible for more than 10 pounds or so. Ask any experienced medical doctor and I'll bet you 49 out of 50 will agree with me. Finding and fixing thyroid trouble doesn't help people lose much weight.

I actually love to find low thyroid hormone in my patients. Most of my treatments don't help people feel as much better as when I can find and fix a low thyroid hormone level.  I usually don't have to remind people to take their thyroid medicine like I have to remind them to take their heart or cholesterol medicines.  They know taking their thyroid pill will make them feel better.  Not many still think it will help them lose weight once they've been on their medicine for very long though.  Calories just count for too much.

Some of my patients are even better at the Internet.  They come to me about their weight but know that the problem is their metabolism or their genes.  Remember the Third Truth?  Calories, either avoiding them or burning them, is more important than your thyroid, your genes and your metabolism.

The thyroid part is pretty easy to prove, and that is why I order so many thyroid tests.  People like proof and I like to give it when I can.  Unfortunately, what I'm going to tell you about metabolism and genes is much harder to prove, but just as true as the rest.  Here goes.


Metabolism is a big word for a big idea.  Metabolism can be thought of as the chemical ways your body breaks apart the food you eat to burn, store, or get rid of as needed.  My favorite medical school class was Physiology.  It was also the hardest and was mostly about one part or another of the human body's metabolism. Scientists can spend their whole careers figuring out one tiny chemical reaction among the many thousands that we lump together and call "metabolism."

This whole complicated thing called metabolism controls two important sides of our food truths. First, it controls how much energy we can squeeze out of our calories. This has to do with chewing, digestion, chemical reactions to make energy, and then storing, moving and using that energy in the right parts of our bodies. Thankfully, this is all automatic for us. I doubt any computer could keep track of all the jobs that our body does without our thinking about it, just to keep us alive and breathing.

Here is the part of metabolism that is closest to the same for every person. This is the part of metabolism most of my patients are thinking about when they blame their weight problem on their metabolism, but our Third Truth says they're wrong.

Unless a person has a serious problem with their intestines not absorbing enough nutrition (which makes them lose weight without meaning to) we all get around 35-40% of the calories we eat turned into energy that we use to live. Anybody from the strongest football linebacker to the wimpiest couch potato among us has about the same level of efficiency.

This is actually what makes the weight loss surgery we talked about earlier work so well for longer than the first few months. At first, people that have had the surgery simply can't eat more than a few mouthfuls without getting a stomachache. As you would expect, they lose weight pretty fast eating only a few mouthfuls a day. The weight loss goes on, though, even after their stomach slowly stretches out to being able to hold a whole meal at once. Why do they still lose weight? Because they had their intestines re-routed to cause the absorbing problem we just talked about. This problem with absorbing is also what turns out to be the biggest issue for them later in life too.

What this means to us it that the Third Truth, that metabolism isn't to blame for my patients' weight problems, is at least mostly true. Everybody that isn't sick or hasn't been re-plumbed inside gets about the same amount of calories out of a Big Mac.

What does change from person to person about their metabolism is also connected to the first two truths. Our example of the pro football player and the couch potato is useful again now. Because the linebacker is a professional athlete and gets paid millions of dollars to keep his body strong and lean, he exercises incredible amounts of time each day and is also very careful about what food he puts into this machine that makes him so rich.

Both what (and not just how much or how many calories) we eat and how much we exercise do matter. Both of these things can make a big difference in how fast we burn the food we take in and the fat we store.

The couch potato and the retired football player will become the size of the couch if they eat what the football star eats everyday just to keep his muscles big. A couch potato (sedentary) average-sized 35-year-old man needs about 2000 calories per day to keep his weight the same, neither gaining nor losing. That linebacker? He needs 6,000 calories per day or more. That's where the "unfairness" I sometimes hear about from people about their metabolism comes in. It is true that some people can eat more than others. The reasons it is true are usually found in how active they are and what they eat, the first two truths.

So who out there with a full-time non-football job and a family can really exercise enough to join the 6,000 calorie club? That linebacker lifts weights 2 hours every day, runs a few miles and puts in a full, sweaty, pounding day of practice to earn his 6,000 calories. You ready?

Since this is way beyond you or me, we have another choice: eating for our own metabolism and gradually trying to speed it up so it helps us lose weight rather than store it around our waists.

# The Fourth Truth

As we started talking about in the last chapter, the 'what' of our eating can make a difference with our metabolisms. We can't make up for 4 hours of heavy exercise every day by changing our eating habits, but we can make a difference. We'll talk about this a lot more later, but the **Fourth Truth** is this: **you are becoming what you eat.**

The couch potato has probably had plenty of potatoes to make him puffy and soft around the middle. Those potatoes will keep him weighted down on the couch, burning calories as slowly as possible. The linebacker eats very differently and it shows. He eats much leaner protein and more complex carbohydrates. He avoids the starches and simple carbohydrates that are so much of the 'typical' American diet.

Eating like this makes him stronger, faster, leaner and has the nice effects of making him feel fuller and burn fat faster too. This Fourth Truth is probably the hardest to want to hear but it might be the most important. We'll come back to it later.

For now, let's sum up what we've talked about before. **The First Truth is that calories count**. How much a person eats is the most important thing anyone can do to affect his or her weight. **The Second Truth is that it is much harder to**

**burn it off than to leave it out.** Once that calorie comes across my tongue and gets swallowed, it's there for the long haul unless I work really hard to get rid of it.

**The Third Truth is that your thyroid, metabolism, and genes don't matter as much as you might wish they did.** Almost everybody gets the same number of calories out of the same foods. Some people do burn calories faster than others, but they were not born that way. Those folks that can burn it fast have worked long and hard to get to that point, and if they ever stop working hard at it, they will go back to the couch potato metabolism the rest of us have to deal with.

**The Fourth Truth is that what I eat really does make me what I am.** Every one of my trillions of cells is made of what I've eaten for lunch, drank at the bar or munched in front of the TV over the years. What I eat makes me and also makes my metabolism faster or slower depending on my choices.

I think each truth fits back into the one before it, so let's have them all in one breath. **What I eat and how much I exercise affects my metabolism, but even my metabolism and my thyroid together aren't nearly as important as how much I eat.**

# Lie Number 1

In the first chapter I started with the lies we are told. Because truth is more important than lies, I went on to talk mostly about some truths I want you to learn and know well. In this chapter we'll return to the lies.

Lies are hard to fight against. Whether just 'a little exaggeration' or 'a real whopper' lies can be hard to pin down and look at. Even though it's hard, finding and pinning down a bunch of food lies is exactly what I want to do with this book.

Some of these lies are just slight distortions of the truth, making them really hard to pin down. When a lie is almost true, I think it is at its strongest. Many of us will want to fight for some of these 'almost true' lies, not because we like lies but because they are old and familiar.

Some of these lies may seem true because we learned them as children, often from our parents or teachers. Remember how young we start to learn our food beliefs? Now, I'm not saying these adults who loved you were trying to lie to you – they probably believed exactly what they were teaching you. The problem is, if Grandma or Mrs. Miller in 2nd grade or whoever else believed and taught you a lie, that lie has an extra strong hold on you because of where you learned it.

Some lies are bold.  The lie we'll start our investigation with is so bold that it is now part of common knowledge and I think you'll have a hard time letting it go, even after we talk it over.  Advertisements, the lunch lady, your mom, 'common sense', maybe even your doctor tell this lie, and boy is it a whopper!

We can easily make a list of truths.  Truth is true and stays true no matter who says it or who hears it.  Lies are much harder to focus on, though.  Everyone hears a lie a little differently.  The 'best' lies even seem to shift around and fit the moment.

That is the power we have to face to get free of the food lies around us.  These lies are powerful, make sense, sound good, sometimes are told by people we trust – but aren't true.

I think that until you can learn to see and fight the lies about your food, you are likely to stay right where you are – stuck at an unhealthy, unfit, and unhappy weight.  My hope is that together we can drag these lies out of the subconscious, out of our habits, out of our high chairs and off the TV.  I think that once you start to see the web of lies surrounding your food, your eyes will open like mine have.

I said we were going to start with a whopper of a lie.  Now, this may not be the most important lie that affects you – in fact, it probably isn't the most important. We are starting with it because of how huge it is, how many people swear its true and how early most of us learn it. It is a great example of the worst kind of lie, the nearly-true, everybody-knows-that kind of lie. If you can really understand this lie – who started it, why it's told, why so many people believe it – then you will be ready to get to the bottom of a whole lot of other food lies.

Ready? **The first lie is… Juice is good for you.**

What? How can that be a lie? Juice **is** good for you, you say. See, I told you it was a whopper. When a lie has been told this many times, it almost becomes true. But it's not true. Juice is **not** good for you or your kids or anyone.

"But what about the vitamins and minerals? The antioxidants?" you say. (I think someone has been watching too many TV commercials.)

Yes, juice has vitamins – but so does the fruit! Yes, juice even has minerals and those antioxidants – but so does the fruit! Know what else juice has? Juice has more calories per ounce than Coke. *Juice has more sugar than soda*. Juice is easier to package and store and ship and sell than fruit. Juice is much sweeter than fruit so it's easier to get kids to like it.

How do any of these things make juice good for you? They don't – it's not! Juice is good for the food and drink companies. Juicing a fruit or vegetable is lots easier than carefully picking it, making sure it looks pretty and doesn't have bruises or worms, then carefully packing and shipping it and hoping you buy it before it spoils. What apple can sit on a shelf as long as a bottle of apple juice? They can really rake in the profits and make you think they care about your health at the same time. Lie!

Do you see how big this lie is? I don't know of another food lie that has been so advertised and so believed as this one. Let me repeat: **Juice is not good for you!**

Fruit is good for you. Fruit has even more of those vitamins, minerals, and antioxidants. Fruit also has fiber and bulk and will fill you up and has way less calories per ounce. Fruit is good, juice is not. It's that simple.

Yes, this is true for vegetable juice too. Radish juice (if you're crazy enough to drink it) has less sugar and fewer calories than orange juice, but the radish is better for you than its juice. Carrots, tomatoes, beets – it's always true that juicing it makes for more calories and less health. Sorry, juice maker companies. Sorry, Tropicana and Welch's and V8. All lies.

Orange juice, apple, grape, even our beloved Juicy Juice ('But it's 100% juice' my patients say) need to go. None of these should be an everyday part of anyone's diet, especially not for kids! A nice treat? A (somewhat) healthier alternative to soda pop? Sure. Something to buy by the gallon and swig with breakfast every morning? No way!

It goes back to our First Truth: Calories Count. Those 8 ounces of OJ (or 12 or 16 or...) every morning will cost you another 20 (or 30 or 40) minutes on the treadmill tonight. How about a glass of water and a vitamin C pill instead? Even better, eat the orange. It has about 1/3 as many calories and is far more filling. The fiber is much better for your digestion than the straight sugar of the juice and the smell of the orange being peeled can actually help you wake up and have a better mood (ask an aromatherapist.)

Some of you are still arguing with me. My patients often do. Sometimes I hear "But it's all-natural." True ... but so are cocaine and arsenic! Just because God put the sugar in it doesn't make it any better for you than if some machine in a factory put the sugar in it.

It's still sugar, still rots your teeth and expands your waist and messes with your intestines. As I see it, you might as well have a Coke and a vitamin pill as drink that glass of orange juice for breakfast. It's about the same thing for your health and waist and probably cheaper for your budget.

Somehow our society has drilled into mothers' heads that good moms give their kids juice for breakfast and snacks and only really bad moms give Coke. What a bunch of hooey! Unfortunately, that hooey runs deep and now 'everybody knows' that juice is good for you. Except now you are starting to re-think this big lie. Keep turning it over in your mind. You really need to understand this lie and the motivation behind the lie being told in the first place if we are going to dig up some of the other lies the food companies want us to believe.

These food lies always have a purpose: <u>selling more whatever</u>. As we start to look for lies, I want you to get better and better at knowing where to look for the lies. By the end of the book, I want your 'lie-detector' to work as well as mine does. If you remember the basic reason why the lies are told — to make more money for whatever company is telling the lies — you have a good start on where to look for the food lies around you.

Some of the lies are bolder than others. Some of the lies seem more 'evil' than others. All of the lies have that one basic purpose: selling. Sometimes the lie is vague and not really said out loud. I'm thinking of the women's magazines that always have 2 headlines, one about how to lose huge amounts of weight quickly and easily and the other about how to make some particularly wonderful dessert. Other lies are right out there in all their misleading, almost-true glory, like the potato chip packages that say in big bold letters "ZERO grams trans-fat!!!" Whether obvious, sneaky, or somewhere in between, the lies are all around us every day. TV, magazines, grocery store aisles, restaurant menus – everywhere.

I said earlier that the 'why' of the lies is my opinion. The basic reason I gave above, making money, should come as no surprise. That's what companies do, if they didn't they wouldn't stay in business. A lot of learning how to find and expose the food lies around you is really just part of being a smart consumer. Advertising will always happen; advertisements will always try to bend the truth to favor whoever paid for them. We shouldn't be surprised.

What I think is going on here is more than just the usual push and pull over truth that you can find in any commercial for a car or toothpaste. Of course, every advertiser claims that their product is going to change your life, clear acne, fix bad breath, help you find true love and make you really, really happy. That's what advertisements do, right? Most adults can see through the car advertisements and tell what is true and what is probably not. I think that for most of us, food lies are much harder to find and see through.

There are plenty of newspaper articles and magazines that use lots of ink and paper to tell you what they think about this or that car or washing machine. For most of the things we buy, a smart consumer can find plenty of help to decide what would be the best to buy. The package or a TV commercial isn't the only place I can find information about a new vacuum cleaner.

Unfortunately, food packaging is more confusing and food costs much less and my need for food is much greater than when I'm shopping for a new computer or cell phone. I'm hungry, tired, and my favorite show starts in 30 minutes. Here I am in aisle 3 looking at the 105 brands of bread my grocery stocks.

How on earth can I tell which one I should buy? Why on earth should I care? Look, that one has a flashing light with a 25 cent coupon dispenser. Cool, it spits out a new coupon every time I wave at it. Oops, now I have 5 coupons, guess I'll get this loaf.

If I even bother to read the packaging, I'm sure I'll feel good about my purchase. Vitamin Fortified! Mom's Favorite! Now with 14 Minerals! Great, glad that was easy. Now, where's the bologna? Off I go, 28 minutes until my show starts.

Again, this is simply my opinion, but I think there is a much more sinister reason for the lies, a reason beyond just selling more and making more money for some company. I told you that the lies are visible, easily found by anyone with the knowledge and motivation to find them. I also said that the 'why' of the lie, other than to make more money for the company that tells it, is my opinion. Well, here is my opinion about the real, deep-down reason companies tell lies in their marketing and on their product packages.

Are you ready for this?

Fat people eat more. Food companies and restaurants want us to be fat so we'll buy more food. Revolting and unfair as it sounds, I really think it's true. A healthy 150 pound woman who is normally active can only eat about 1,500 calories a day without steadily getting heavier. If that woman can be tricked into eating 300 extra calories per day (one candy bar or two Cokes or an extra big handful of chips), in five years she'll weigh close to 200 pounds. By that time, her stomach has stretched and her daily calorie needs are 500 calories higher, meaning she will buy more food.

Fifty years from now, I think there will be hearings in Congress over the conspiracy against consumers by the food companies. It will look a lot like our current rage against the tobacco companies for lying to us and our kids for the last 80 years. Tobacco companies intentionally lied about how addictive their product was and worked to make it more addictive, all while hiding the fact that they knew tobacco killed people.

I think food companies know how addictive their additives are, they know how misleading their advertisements and menus are, they know that we are getting fatter and fatter and eating more and more, **and they planned it that way**.

See why I'm mad?  Lying to sell something is almost the American way.  Lying to intentionally hurt someone so you can sell more of something is way beyond American.  It's disgusting.

Enough preaching for the moment, let's move on to another lie.

# Lie number 2

Drive-thrus, vending machines, gas station soda fountains – I think I'm within 2 minutes of a refreshing 44 ounce cup of something sweet, cold, and fizzy all day. It quenches my thirst, wakes me up, gives me energy and makes me feel good. For a lot of us, the sound of the pull tab or lid being opened or the gurgle of the soda fountain giving out its cold drink is almost heavenly.

Some of the lies I write about are more personal than others. This is probably my biggest weakness. I used to joke that I had a legal coke addiction. It was true and I still love to hear the sounds a can of Coke makes when I open and drink it. At one point I even figured out a way to have a vending machine in my office just so I had easier access to my daily Coke 'fix'.

Yeah, it was just a wee bit hypocritical, telling people that they needed to eat healthier, lose weight, blah blah blah all while a big red Coca-Cola machine sat glowing in my office waiting room.

Americans are social eaters. One of the most neighborly things you can do is share a meal with someone. Sharing a drink feels almost as bonding. I think that's why the old jingle "Have Coke and a smile" has its power. Sharing something to eat or drink with someone is good for us and for our relationships.  Many families keep something quick and convenient around to share just for this purpose.

Remember our math in the first chapter?  One can of Coke has 150 calories which takes 30 minutes to walk off.  This mix of fizzy water and sugar that I sometimes crave so much is absolutely loaded with the emptiest of calories, but come on, one can won't hurt.  **The second lie is … Soda pop is harmless.**

There are a couple of lies buried in this one and I want to dig them up and look at them in the light.  One of these lies is something nearly every food company is guilty of: up-sizing. Looking at old packaging, I wonder if The Coca-Cola Company wasn't the first to try this lie out.

Have you seen those cute old Coke bottles?  Those of us that are old enough remember the old-style vending machines that dispensed the little 8 ounce glass bottle with the pry-off cap.  Those machines even had a place to pry off the cap, so you could get that first drink right away.

That 8 ounce bottle was sold for a quarter in my earliest memories, though I know it was a dime not long before my childhood and a nickel before that.  Think of the ratio of how much it cost the company to mix the Coke to put in the bottle versus making the bottle and shipping it to where a customer could get their hands on it.  Someone very smart realized that the Coke was the cheap part, so why not sell bigger bottles of Coke for slightly more money and have a bigger profit margin?

It has been years since we could easily find the 8 ounce bottle of Coke, but the nutrition information on the can or bottle you buy still calculates a serving based on that little old 8 ounce bottle. Of course, now a 12-ounce can is the smallest common size you can get, but what about the 20 ounce or the 24 ounce or the liter or the 2 liter? Each larger size is a better and better profit margin for the company and every size says '100 calories' at the top of the nutrition label. Even if someone is interested enough to look, they're liable to be misled by that old lie.

The up-sizing of a "serving" of Coke has taken years, but what most people think of as one Coke is at least the 20 ounce bottle and maybe even the 32 ounce fountain drink. What I think of as one Coke and what someone else thinks of as one Coke can be very different, but whatever size we think of for "one" Coke is bigger than the 8 ounce serving size. Depending on the amount of ice you get, one of the handy 44 ounce sizes my local convenience store sells for 99 cents will have 400- 500 calories! That's right, 3 hours of fast walking to get rid of that Super-Sized Coke from McDonald's or the gas station. Care to calculate the effort required to burn off the whole McDonald's meal or the Big

Grab bag of chips that tastes so good with my little afternoon pick-me-up drink?

This is where America's weight problem, many of my patients' weight problem, maybe even your weight problem comes from. Calories that we never really think about sneak in with our little afternoon snack and pretty soon, stretchy pants.

I know it's unfair. I know it's not easy to resist or even to see these lies and tricks. I also know **there is no possible way to eat like an American and not get fat.** This is exactly why 2 out of every 3 American adults are at least 30 pounds overweight. Worse, 1 out of 3 Americans is at least 60 pounds overweight and has the health problems to prove it.

I told you before that there are at least a couple of lies involved in the whole soda pop scheme. Up-sizing is certainly the most serious and the most intentional lie the companies are telling us, making larger and larger sizes to increase their profit margin and our waist lines. The other lie is much more subtle and a little harder to figure out, but makes the up-sizing lie even more serious.

The other lie is actually our brain's fault, not something dreamed up by the food and drink companies, but wow does it make those soda pop calories a problem.

Everyone has a food thermostat, a sensor that tells them when they are getting hungry, when they are really hungry, and when that hunger has gotten to the point that their body really has to have something to eat or else. These thermostats are very finicky and easy to ruin by habit or upbringing or bad food choices, but the thermostat is meant to keep us from starving to death. Hundreds of years ago, food was much harder to get than it is today. Storing food was very difficult before refrigerators and freezers and almost everything had to be made from scratch just before it was eaten. Many years before that, our ancestors didn't even have the ability to prepare complicated meals or store grains and vegetables and had to actually find the food before they could do whatever preparing they knew how to do.

All this means that it could take several hours or longer just to get ready to eat, so that food thermostat had to give plenty of warning that it was time to start thinking about food and finding some to get ready. Without this early warning system, our ancestors wouldn't have had time to find and fix their food before their bodies started acting up over being starved.

While it was good for us humans many years ago and allowed us to survive long enough to invent refrigerators and restaurants, that food thermostat is a big part of our weight problem now.  We will talk about this food thermostat again later, but the part that has to do with soda pop is still buried in the thermostat idea.

This thermostat is also how our body signals the need for something to drink or that we are thirsty.  This means that hunger can actually be thirst, but if the thermostat shut off once we took a drink of water, our ancestors might have starved, so it generally doesn't shut off until we have actually eaten.  When the only thing there is to drink is water, no problem.  When our drinks have more calories per ounce than some foods, big problem.

Here is the subtle lie about soda pop, one caused by our bodies but used by the food and restaurant companies to sell more of everything.  Most people have a food thermostat that is not at all satisfied by the calories in a drink.  This means that **no matter how many refills the restaurant gives away or how big McDonald's up-sizes their drinks, it won't affect how much food people buy or eat.**

Did you get that?  Water is the same as soda pop, is the same as juice, is the same as beer to your appetite.  The extra calories in our drinks are truly extra, because our bodies don't count them towards telling us when to stop eating.  This is a serious problem, folks!  Those calories are there, those calories stick to our waists like any other calories, but our stomach and appetites can't figure it out.

Like I said, those food thermostats are finicky and often out of whack anyway, but add to that the fact that they just don't register the calories of our drinks and WHAMO, we have a problem.

These two lies about soda pop are big enough that together they are probably the worst single weight-producing problem most of my patients face. Soda pop is exactly what most of us crave, with quick, energy-giving sugar combined with a taste, sound and feel that are hard to get out of other food and drinks. Worse, soda pop is also sold in huge sizes for cheap prices and our appetites often don't even realize that we just had 500 calories in that super-size soda pop.

If you don't struggle with soda pop, count yourself lucky, because many of us do and let me tell you, it is hard to stop. But stop we must if we ever want to get control of our calories and our weights, because soda pop is a big part of our bigness problem. We'll talk about it more later, but even diet soda pop is a problem, even though a huge cup of Diet whatever has no calories itself. The most commonly used artificial sweetener actually makes us eat more and probably leads to more weight gain than just drinking the real thing! Terrible!

Let's get back to our Four Truths again. We've been looking in-depth at food lies and have so far covered 2 of the biggest and most important: **Juice is good for you** and **Soda pop is harmless.**

I don't want lies and conspiracy theories to wear us out, so let's review the Truths again, clear our minds, and talk about the positive. Do you remember them?

Truth One: My calories count

Truth Two: I can't exercise my way to weight loss

Truth Three: My metabolism is not to blame

Truth Four: I am what I eat

The first two Lies are important because of Truth One. Unless you deep down believe me about calories counting, it will be hard to take the Juice and Soda Pop lies seriously enough.

# Counting those Calories that Count

Before we move on to revealing more lies, I'd like you to take a minute and a calculator and learn just how many calories are recommended for you, based on your age, sex, weight, and activity level. **This calorie limit is a number you need to know and take to heart if you want to conquer your weight and waist.** The equation used to find this number is almost a hundred years old and just to make matters worse, it's in metric. It's called the Harris-Benedict Equation and doctors actually use this for very sick patients to decide how many calories to feed them (usually through a tube) while the patient is in bed sick. It can be adjusted based on the patient's type of illness and whether they can do any physical activity.

Here I've made the equation much simpler by using age categories and converting to pounds and leaving out height. This leaves a range of about 125 calories higher or lower for any one particular person, so the number you get could vary from the actual number you would get with the real equation by about 125 calories higher or lower. If you're a real nerd like me, you can Google search the name of the equation and do the precise calculation. For the rest of us, here are the approximate calculations:

**Men**  18-29 years old

    **Calories = 6.8 x weight in pounds + 690**

**Men**  30-59 years old

    **Calories = 5.2 x weight in pounds + 870**


**Women**  18-29 years old

    **Calories = 6.7 x weight in pounds + 490**

**Women**  30-59 years old

    **Calories = 3.7 x weight in pounds + 840**


These numbers then have to be multiplied by your activity level.  This factor is less agreed upon than the first equation, so we'll have to make do with an estimate.  If you have a desk job and get no daily organized exercise, multiply your number by 1.2.  If you have a physical job like construction or landscaping, multiply your number by 1.4.  If you get at least 30 minutes of sweaty exercise 3 or 4 days per week, multiply your number by 1.4

Most people will calculate something between 1,500 and 2,500 calories.  **This is the total number of calories needed**

**for the day and every calorie you eat, drink or chew on** (check out the calories in your favorite piece of gum) **counts toward this number.**

When you realize that a Large Coke, Large fries and Quarter Pounder with Cheese at McDonald's is 1,350 calories (that's using only 2 packets of ketchup), you can tell how easy it is to go WAY over your daily calorie need.  It's easy to see why 2 out of every 3 Americans are overweight.  How about a full-day typical American diet of quick and simple American take-out?

Let's pick average items, not the most unhealthy but rather menu choices that seem like a 'better, healthier' meal. Starbuck's for breakfast, Burger King for lunch, and Chinese take-out for supper.  Who hasn't eaten this way when pressed for time?  It's not even that expensive and might be cheaper than buying the ingredients to make healthy, homemade meals.

At Starbuck's, I hit the drive-thru for a quick breakfast, avoid the sell of the day ("would you like to try our gourmet cinnamon roll with that?") and stick to what seems like a healthier choice: a Grande (medium) Cappuccino with a wheat bagel and light cream cheese (140 calories for the cappuccino from the Starbuck's website, about 350 calories for the bagel and cream cheese based on estimates from other websites, since Starbuck's won't count food calories for us on their website.)

For lunch, a co-worker offers to pick up Burger King, not my favorite, but I'll make do. I ask for the Tender Crisp chicken sandwich and onion rings, thinking the chicken is better for me than that Whopper everyone talks about being so fattening, plus the onion rings have some vegetables in them, right? Oh yeah, and get me a large Coke too, that should hold me through the afternoon fade. So let's see, that's 800 calories for the sandwich, 450 for the medium rings, and 400 for the Coke. So far I'm just over 2000 calories for the day and it's only one o'clock.

That's my whole day's worth of food, finished before I've been awake 6 hours. What about my afternoon pick-me-up snack, supper at the Chinese place and maybe a bowl of ice cream for bedtime snack? Boy did I need a mint or two after those onion rings for lunch, plus this morning I needed two more cups of the office coffee to keep me awake. It tastes so bad I needed plenty of that Hazelnut creamer just to choke it down. Somebody brought Dunkin Donuts, but I resisted and only had three or four of those donut holes with my cup of coffee -- both cups, that is.

Do you see all this? I've just crossed 4000 calories for the day, done with best intentions and even trying to pay attention to what I eat. I at least noticed the snacks, I didn't eat at any buffets where no one can count calories but everyone loosens their belt and since its winter, the ice cream place down the road is still closed so there was no late-night parfait run.

No one can get away with this for long before it catches up to them and hangs 30 or 50 or 100 pounds around their waists. No one. That's why I'm writing all this, that's hopefully why you're reading all this, to change our behaviors and habits, to open our eyes to what we're putting into our mouths.

Remember our calculations above? How even ten extra calories a day for a year add up to a pound of fat? These little splurges add up just like the financial costs of them add up over years and can reach into the many thousands of dollars. David Bach wrote a book about the $5 latte, calculating that if that $5 is saved daily for 30 years, you could have almost **half a million** dollars.

The same calculations for that latte should be done for its calories. Starbucks 'Tall' (meaning small) regular latte has 180 calories. If I enjoy one every day for a year, that is over 65,000 calories and **nearly 2 million calories** over the same 30 years. All that from a cup of coffee!!??!!

The extra pounds people gain in their twenties and thirties that lead to health problems in their forties and fifties can all be avoided by skipping those little sources of daily calories that slip past our notice.  We just need to learn to notice those sneaking calories and make sure too many don't sneak past our lips.

# Lie number 3

**You should get your money's worth.**  I'm writing this during the biggest economic slump since the Great Depression. Money is on everyone's mind.  Can I afford gas at $2.50 (or $3.50, or...)?  Will I get laid off?  Will my company even be in business in a year?

In this sort of economy, money concerns are at the top of most of our worry lists and finding a good deal is not just fun and satisfying (ask a dedicated garage-saler) but also important.  It seems like most advertisements aim right at this fear, emphasizing how this or that product is such a bargain.

Nowhere is this bargain finding more obvious than with our food.  Ninety-nine cent 'Value Menus', super-sizing meals, jumbo pizzas, all-you-can-eat, coupons, kids-eat-free -- the list goes on.  It seems like there is a bargain on food at every restaurant, down every food aisle, even at the gas station Qwik-Mart: Buy one 20 ounce Coke, get one free! (That will be 500 calories, please.)

Now don't get me wrong.  I like sales as much as the next person - ask my wife how often I'll drive way out of the way to save a nickel a gallon on gas.  I'm glad to find my favorite 100% whole wheat bread on sale 2-for-1 or 50 cents off my favorite six-pack of beer.  What gets me steamed are the other kinds of sales, the ones that get people to buy the less nutritious, higher calorie, bigger serving substitute as a way to 'save money.'

Grocery stores seem to do this in rotation, sometimes having the 'good stuff' on sale, other times the not so good stuff. Maybe they're just trying to get rid of back stock and prevent food from spoiling before it's sold. Whatever the reason, frozen pizza, macaroni and cheese, and Hamburger Helper are terrible for families trying to make their money stretch and I cringe to see them on sale. I am enough of a realist to know that I won't talk stores into not putting this stuff on sale let alone not stocking it at all - unless we change how we buy food. Like I said earlier, only when Americans stop buying garbage will stores stop selling it.

As upset as I get in the grocery aisle, restaurants make me even angrier. Groceries are at least labeled so if I really want to (and I do) I can figure out just what I'm eating and make better choices. How many restaurants will tell you what's in their food and how many calories you're paying for? New York City has started to require this, which has really ticked off restaurants. They seem to think that if people know that such and such pasta dish, salad and garlic bread costs over 4000 calories, then maybe folks won't order it so often. Of course I think that would be great!

But unless you live in the Big Apple or go to one of a handful of restaurants that will actually tell you how badly their food sticks to your waist, you're on your own to figure out which is the better choice between foods or restaurants. Scientists have studied how well we do figuring this out on our own, and let me tell you, it's not pretty!

People are <u>terrible</u> at guessing how many calories are in a dish or which dish is healthier or even how many calories their bodies need. When I read some of this research I realized how much people need to learn about food and I got motivated to write this book.

All of us, you and me and Grandma and the second grade teacher are born without even a clue about food and nutrition. We don't have any healthy instincts about food and can't rely on common sense either. These scientists have proven over and over again that **without extra learning and effort, people will pick the wrong foods in the wrong amounts every time**.

The good news is that I personally know people who have taken this knowledge and changed their lives. They have lost weight, gained energy and restored their health simply by learning and using new food habits like we are talking about. I want that for you too!

The sad truth is that it is cheaper and easier in 21$^{st}$ century America to eat poorly than it is to eat healthy. Buying and fixing healthy food is harder than hitting the drive-thru and it always will be. I want you to open your mind to what 'getting your money's worth' should mean.

If filling your belly in the quickest and cheapest way possible is what you mean by this, then McDonald's will be happy and stay in business. I want people to think about their lives, not just their stomachs, though. How is a $50,000 heart attack surgery getting your money's worth? Is needing to buy a new wardrobe every year to help hide the love handles getting your money's worth? Maybe not being able to keep up with your kids because of your weight is the price you are willing to pay to save on groceries, but I hope not.

Folks, this is huge. This may be the most important thing I've got to say, so listen up.

**Your life and your health are the only really valuable possessions you have.**

Almost everything else can be replaced or repaired. Not so easy to replace or repair the amazing machine you tool around in all day. Your body will <u>always</u> treat you the way you treat it. If I put watered-down gas in my car's tank and let a tire run flat and refuse to 'waste money' on changing the oil, how well do you think my car will run?

Like a teenager's body, at first everything will run just fine. Fourteen-year-olds can usually get away with eating absolutely anything and still have great energy. They can stay awake all night at a pajama party, stuffing their face with pizza and Coke, and not get heartburn or even a headache.

What if I make a forty year old spend a few nights like this? How well will my body hold up to this sort of treatment? How well would you hold up? Once our cars (and bodies) have a few years and miles on them, they must be taken care of or they will break down – guaranteed. Much early aging is caused by what we do to ourselves. All of our weight gain is caused by what we do to ourselves

Everybody has heard "You get what you pay for." My dad used this to teach me about buying well-made things, not just the cheapest or most convenient. My favorite singer Dave Matthews has turned this on its head with the line "You pay for what you get." His approach makes my point about food much better than the common sense version does.

I do pay for what I eat and will keep paying for what I eat. This is really important to learn and believe and know down deep. Knowing that <u>food has consequences</u> is a big deal and I want you to learn that well.

What I choose, what you choose to eat makes a world of difference to your body, your health, your weight. The fatty, full of cholesterol lunch that is so cheap at McDonald's has consequences, today and tomorrow and for years to come.

The high fat content will make me sleepy in the next hour as my body actually takes blood away from vital organs to try to digest this meal. The starch in the bun and the fries and the sugar in the soda pop will give me immediate energy and also a guaranteed sugar crash in about 2 hours, probably making me feel hungry again even though my intestines will still be hard at work trying to digest the rest of it.

By that evening or the next day, I'll probably have gas and diarrhea from the strain that kind of eating puts on my digestion. I'll definitely have thicker blood with a much higher fat content as my liver tries to cope with all the fat. My liver cells will package all that fat and float it along my bloodstream to where I store it (for me, it's unfortunately in my love handles) though that process takes a few more days.

What about the cholesterol and the preservatives? Here is the part that may never go away. The same blood vessels that carry the fat from my liver to my love handles actually get damaged by such high fat content and some of that fat seeps into the lining of the veins and arteries. If that happens in the arteries around my heart then I've just gotten a little bit closer to the heart attack coming down the road.  Nice thought, huh?

All of these results from one meal at a fast food place?  You bet.  Maybe now you can see why I so rarely eat this stuff.  Yes, it's convenient and cheap.  But I <u>know</u> what food like this does to my body and I know there's nothing cheap or convenient about fixing the damage it can do.  What I want is for my patients and my readers to know all this as well as I do and then to change where and what they eat.  That is the key to health now and in the future.

# Lie Number 4

**"I can't change."** For some of us, this is the strongest lie in the world. Yes, it's a lie, even when it's that strong, but realizing and learning to live free of this lie is really hard. It's also really important.

One of my most important jobs as a family doctor is helping people learn to fight this lie. Folks really get held back by this, thinking "this is just how I am" or "this is how all my family is." Family genes, personal choices, life twists and turns all make us who we are today but none of these have to keep us that way.

After years of watching, talking to and learning from my patients I have become convinced that we are free. **The lie "I can't change" isn't true because we are free.** Humans can always change; people can always turn around and become different.

For some people the possible change that feels impossible is about their smoking. For others it is about their couch potato habits. For many, it's their food choices, food addictions, and their slowly growing waistline. No matter what someone's issue or addiction or hang-up is, I really, truly believe it is possible to change.

Is it easy? Heck no. Is it likely? Not if they don't really want to. But is it humanly possible? Absolutely. That's why I'm getting carpal tunnel by writing all this and killing trees to print it. **Because people can change, because you can change and because the effort is worth it.**

One of the most famous organizations for change is Alcoholics Anonymous. They have helped people make a very hard change for many years. Most people have heard of their philosophy called The 12 Steps. These steps are the most basic level of learning for someone who wants to be free of alcohol. Some people are so addicted to bad food choices that they need a 12-step program to be free of their health and weight problems.

If that is you then please get the help you need. Overeaters Anonymous, Food Addicts Anonymous and other recovery groups exist to help you. Get on the Internet and find a local group and go.

No matter who we are and how much of a problem we might have, a version of the First Step is crucial. The original wording is of course about alcohol, but psychologists will tell you that "The first step is admitting you have a problem." This is truly the first step in any change and the place we have to start.

Only once I see that something is wrong can I start to make a change. If my buddy doesn't tell me I have toothpaste smeared on my lip, I won't know to wipe it off. If my wife doesn't tell me my shirt and slacks don't really match, I'm going to look silly all day. If I don't tell my patients about their weight or cholesterol or sugar problem, they may not know that they need to change.

Once I know a problem exists, then it's in my hands. Hopefully I'll get the toothpaste wiped off or my shirt changed before I embarrass myself.

# Lie number 5

**"But I don't eat that much."**  Wow, here's a doozy.  If this list of lies was a popularity contest, this would probably be number 2 (the one about juice is still the most common.)  I hear this every day as a doctor and have spent years trying to get a handle on it.

I know my patients aren't intentionally lying to me and they're not stupid either.  So how do I jive this with the Truths?  The Truths make it pretty plain that I believe weight is <u>always</u> a calorie issue, I won't believe my patients are dumb or liars, and yet so many of them are overweight and tell me they don't eat that much.  Quite a conundrum.

I saved this lie for this far down our list because I think it is so heavily affected by the lies and truths we've already looked at.  On the surface it seems pretty simple, but really it is a very hard-to-fix problem with how people think about their food and eating habits.

When I was new to being a doctor, I would often try to argue people out of their beliefs about how much they eat.  The Truths are true and I've known them for about as long as I've been a doctor, so I needed to make people see the truth, right?  Let me tell you, it's hard to argue someone into a new point of view as part of a 15-minute appointment.

Besides the time factor, I had a few other difficulties winning this argument.

For one, most people can't be argued into or out of *anything*, let alone something this big. Have you ever tried to argue someone into liking your baseball team better than theirs? How about going door to door before the big election, trying to argue folks into voting for your candidate? It's hard to do; in case you've never tried, take it from me.

Anything folks care about at all, especially if they have emotions tied up in why they think the way they do, is near and dear to their heart. I might as well try to argue them into believing my mom is better than their mom as try to win an argument with my patients about how much they eat.

Like I said, for years I tried to argue folks into taking my view (maybe I haven't stopped – isn't this book one long argument?) I eventually settled on a brief little speech meant to keep me and my patients friends and not waste a whole appointment bickering. It went something like this:

> I hear your frustration, Ms. Brown, and wish I had a different answer for you, but I don't. No one can gain weight without eating too many calories – it's simple math and it affects everyone. I'd like you to take my food diary challenge – I've never lost when a

patient has taken me up on it.  If you write down everything you eat and drink for the next 2 weeks and bring it back to me, I promise we can find the extra calories that are sneaking in on you and then we can fix this.

As you can guess, not many people took me up on this challenge.  It sounds hard (it's not – try it for just 2 days and you'll see) and it sounds risky (it is – people risk losing their favorite excuse), but those who did it always found out Truth Number 1 by personal example.  We always found the extra calories because they are always there.

It really is impossible to gain weight without eating more than your body needs.  I am always excited when someone takes their new knowledge and changes their life by losing the weight that has hounded them for years.  The amazing success of these people always kept me hoping that the next person, my next patient, might be another one who believed me, took my challenge, and then took control of their food and won.

It was this steady stream of conversations over the years that lead to me sitting down to write this book.  My hope is that if I could give each patient a crash course in medical school nutrition then many more would learn what needs to be done and how simple (not easy, just simple) it really is and finally change their health for the better.  That's what this book is – everything I've learned about food and nutrition and weight loss all in one spot.

As my practical nutrition knowledge grew and as more research into the subject became available, I realized I had more than my usual speech to give people when they said "but I don't eat that much." Every time someone took my food diary challenge, I learned another calorie pitfall people can fall into.

For one person it's soda pop, another it's juice – which is why these 2 lead the way in my list of lies. Others found a forgotten bowl of late night ice cream or potato chips. Still others learned the hard way how many calories are in their favorite café mocha latte or morning donut.

I've found carrot dip, chips and salsa, sweet tea and even weight loss drinks to be the problem. Anything that has calories but doesn't really seem like it does can be the problem.


Some scientists have done really good studies about people and their food that have helped me understand more about this issue too. Now, before we get into this, we all need to agree that I'm not trying to offend anyone or accuse anyone of lying. Many of these scientists have said that they were surprised how mad people got when they found out the results of the testing that had been done on them.

First about the research:  no one was dissected or put in a test tube or anything creepy or weird like that.  This research was all done just by watching people.  The cool (for me) part is that these scientists were so clever figuring out what to watch people do and where to watch them in order to give us good information about how we pick foods.

There has been research about almost everything you can think of to do with food, though most of it is just taste-testing and is how many of our foods have come to be so bad for us.  The problem with the bad-for-you food is that it's good.  By using taste-improving additives and ingredients, choosing the right color and feel to their foods, even figuring out who would probably buy their food and where they most likely eat it, companies have figured out how to make people want and buy more of their products. That's not the kind of research I'm interested in though. From my angle, they're the bad guys, trying to get you and me and the mailman to eat more and to eat more often.

The kind of research we're going to talk about here is meant to help us understand why so many of us struggle with our weight and learn how we can fight back.  Perfect, huh?

Unfortunately, there isn't nearly as much money put into this type of research as the other, 'bad guy' kind. No restaurant or food company is going to pay for research into helping people eat less, so this kind of scientist has a harder time getting money for her projects.

Some of these scientists have persevered and done their research anyway, so let's find out what they've learned. These experiments were mostly done on normal people in normal kitchens, dining rooms, and living rooms with either cameras or two-way mirrors installed so the scientists could watch and measure what and when and how much people ate.

Every person in these studies was a volunteer, often joining an experiment about food because of their own struggles with weight and nutrition. Many of the people in these experiments also had a face-to-face conversation with the scientists running the experiment about what the experiment found.

In the last 20 years, science has discovered a lot about our appetites and food habits. What these scientists haven't found is even one person who gained weight without excess calories. Not one. I think this is why the scientists talk about people getting mad at them at the end of the experiments, because most of us want our favorite excuse to be true. "But I don't eat that much" has <u>never</u> turned out to be true.

So what gives? How do so many people feel the same way about their weight and appetite? These experiments are much more about the mental part of our eating than about the physical part of eating. Remember my medical school class with all the chemical reactions? These scientists have proven the chemical side of digestion and calories beyond any doubt. The psychology (or subconscious or "head") part of what, when, why, and how much we eat is harder to figure out, more interesting, and much more useful for those of us trying to learn new habits.

As I said above much of this research has been done by a small group of dedicated scientists. I want to talk about 3 different results these scientists have uncovered. The first of these is about how well people estimate the number of calories they eat and the size of a portion of food. The second result is about how much people exercise compared to how much they think they exercise. The third is about simple but very clever ways these scientists have come up with to trick the brain into wanting to eat less.


In 1992, Steven Heymsfield, M.D., published a fascinating experiment about how well people estimate what they eat.

His research showed that among people with a long-term weight problem, every one of them estimated the number of calories eaten daily at <u>half</u> of what they actually ate. This means that these overweight and obese people would honestly tell themselves or their doctor that they counted their calories and only ate 1,000 a day. When those calories were carefully counted by someone else, each of them actually ate <u>over 2,000 calories a day</u>.

This is exactly what we have been talking about and a perfect example of "hidden calories" that so easily sneak up and bite us in the butt. These people who agreed to let Dr. Heymsfield study their eating habits were chosen because of their lifelong problems with being overweight and their strong interest in dieting and losing weight. These folks weren't lazy or dumb or unmotivated, just frustrated.

When I read this study I became even more driven to educate my patients about better eating and to write this book. I want to help educate many more frustrated and discouraged people. This is strong scientific proof that our appetites cannot be trusted. I think most of us have a food IQ of about 25 which means "profoundly retarded."

"But Dr. Marcotte," you're saying right now, "does that mean it's hopeless? Does that mean I have no hope of learning my food and losing weight?"

Far from it! We are pretty much stuck with our normal IQ but no one is stuck with their food IQ. That's the whole point of buying and reading this book. You have already raised your food IQ a lot, and the more you learn and know about your food and choices the better your chances of being set free from your weight problem.

Dr. Heymsfield and his colleagues also investigated how well people estimated their activity level or how many calories they burned through exercise. He found that this number was way off too, making the calorie problem even worse. People tend to think that they eat much less and exercise much more than they really do.

Did you see those numbers? Folks eat 1,000 calories more than they think and exercise 300 calories less than they think! That's 1,300 calories a day difference! No wonder so many people are frustrated about their weight. Here is the reason many people truly think they eat 1,000 calories a day and exercise at least 300 more calories off and yet are slowly gaining weight instead of steadily losing.

Doctors know exactly what happens when a person eats 1,000 calories a day and exercises 300 of them off – they end up in the hospital. Nobody can do that without losing weight at a dangerous rate and getting very ill. This is a problem: what I know would happen and what some of my patients think should happen in the same circumstances are very, very different.

Apparently the people in this experiment were just as upset about the results as you probably are right now. No one likes to hear that they're wrong let alone that they're usually wrong. But that is exactly what the science of diet and eating has proven over and over again. I don't know how many of the people in his experiments believed Dr. Heymsfield or whether they all walked away refusing to believe.

My patients have the same choice when I tell them something that goes against what they want to believe and so do you. You can pooh-pooh this and choose to believe that you are an exception to the rule and continue as things are. But I think a better option might be to keep your mind open and keep trying to learn new habits so you can make new choices. Keep reading and keep thinking about this as we move on to talk about another set of experiments.

James Levine, MD published an interesting experiment that measured how much people move and found some shocking facts. All of us know someone who seems to eat and eat but never gets fat. When they are confronted with this unfairness, they usually claim 'a fast metabolism,' the rest of us grumble about that being unfair and we all move on.  Now we just read about Dr. Heymsfield's research proving that folks don't have the slow metabolism they think they do, so what gives?

Dr. Levine's study measured every movement every second of the day in 20 people who got no regular exercise. Remember, it's no fair comparing yourself to the professional linebacker who works out 4 hours a day.  This experiment picked 'regular' folks, too busy or tired or unmotivated to work out.  What Dr. Levine did that was unique was find folks that were couch potatoes but that had different body weights, some normal weight and some overweight.  None of these folks had any special instructions, just to go about their day as usual.

Each of them wore a special full-body set of underwear that measured every muscle and recorded it for the scientists. When the information was collected, Dr. Levine and his team found out exactly why those skinny couch potatoes stayed skinny.  Just by doing their normal activities, the skinny folks burned over 300 calories more per day than the fluffy folks did!

'Now that is unfair,' you say.  'See, I knew some folks had better metabolisms.'

Well, wait a minute. This experiment wasn't measuring metabolism, like the last one. Dr. Levine knew that part has already been proven and that folks don't have abnormal metabolisms. What Dr. Levine found was how much more some people move compared to others <u>without meaning to</u>.

That's right; those 300+ calories were all burned without any exercise. This is what some people call 'nervous energy.' These lucky folks fidget their way to a normal weight without diet or exercise.

The good news for you and me is that this habit of extra movement can be learned. Some people are just wired to be on the move, others to move more slowly and conserve energy. Learning to keep yourself moving can be the equivalent of dieting for those 300 calories. Without joining the gym, people can learn to burn more fat and calories.

Toe-tapping, finger twiddling, jumping up for spontaneous walks, even sitting up straight without leaning into the chair back are all examples of the movements people made in this experiment. These are movements you and I can learn to copy and make a habit of doing. Combine 300 extra calories burned here with another 300 calories avoided in snacks or beverages and suddenly you could be losing weight at a pound a week!

See, calories count and it doesn't even hurt.

Before we learned about the science about food and eating, we were talking about 'hidden calories.' Foods that seem healthy or that are easy to forget or seem like they don't count can all be 'hidden calories.' In fact, any calorie that a person can't or won't see could be called 'hidden,' though some calories are much better hidden than others.

The better a calorie is hidden, the more likely that some food company is intentionally misleading us. If people are kept in the dark about calories, they won't worry about buying drinks or snacks or coffee or a morning donut, because "it's so little, it doesn't matter." I want my patients and my readers to know how much it does matter. That's the only way to fight this lie.

It's not easy. If you want to learn your way through the lie "But I don't eat that much," it will take paying attention to things you've always ignored and learning new habits. I don't think it takes becoming a vegetarian or food Nazi though. What you have to do is give some time and attention to making new habits and then to open your eyes to what you are buying and eating.

Any habit takes about 3 months to make and once you've made these new habits, it's easy. Seriously. If you'll spend the time and energy to learn your food and care about what you buy and eat, you will find that it works. You will lose weight and keep it off and it will become easier and easier until it is automatic.

Then, dear reader, you will have won. You will have the knowledge and the power and the habits to make a healthy weight yours for life.

That's why the lie we tell ourselves about how much we eat is so important for us to conquer. It is probably the most emotionally difficult lie on the list for most of us. **The deep down realization that "I do eat too much and only I can fix this" is both very important and very hard to swallow.**

It's important because this is where the power I mentioned really comes from. It's hard because this is taking personal responsibility for what family, teachers, friends, TV and advertisements have taught you over the years. I know it's not fair but it's the only option.

No one plans to learn lies as a little kid, so having to take responsibility for those lies as an adult is truly unfair. So, admit life is unfair then take this lie by the horns and win!

# About Reading Packages

A big part of being a family doctor is paying attention to the little things. I do that pretty well. If you ask my wife she might tell you I pay a little too much attention to detail sometimes. When it comes to food, though, this is a good habit to get into.

Thirty years ago, we had no way of really knowing what we were putting into our bodies. More recently, the federal government has started paying attention to how heavy we are all getting and made rules about labeling food that are at least a step in the right direction. You may have seen this labeling, though you have to be looking for it to find it. The front of the package you see in the grocery is fair game for advertising and may say almost anything.

"Zero grams trans-fat" "Whole grains for your heart" "Now 30% leaner" "Lose weight and feel great"

You know what those labels say. The shelves are packed, there are little coupon dispensers and sale cards and bright lights everywhere, you're tired and hungry and just want to get some groceries and get home to dinner. The last thing most people do is turn over the colorful, pretty package and look at the scientific stuff on the back.

Problem is, that's what I plan to teach you to do. The way the laws are made, this is about the only part of the package that has to tell you the truth. Unfortunately even here the food companies have figured out ways to lie and mislead. We'll talk about those ways a little later. For right now, the most important thing is remembering to turn the package over and look at the Nutrition Label.

The law that makes food companies do this also says what has to be shown and where. That at least makes our learning a little easier, since once you learn where to find the information on one package, you can be sure that the next package will have (almost) the same information .

Go to your cupboard or pantry and pick up some packaged grocery item. Fresh foods generally don't have to list this, so a banana won't tell you what you want to know, but the banana pudding next to it will. Some practice will make this label reading seem easier and easier until it's second nature for you like it is for me. Now is when we have to start looking for the lies I talked about earlier, though.

Some law made the food companies tell you how many calories, carbohydrate and fat grams they used. What that law didn't do was make them list the quality or the quantity of the ingredients they used. We'll get to reading the label for quality later when we talk about the Fourth Truth in depth. For now, I want to focus on the biggest lie companies are allowed to tell in that Nutrition Label.

Even here, they aren't really lying, but dang if they aren't trying to mislead. Above the line that draws your eye and leads you to the calories and other stuff you'd think are important, are two even more important and very misleading pieces of information.

As an example, I'll go back to that can of Coke we've talked about before. Curious Coke drinkers out there may have already turned around the label and read what it says. These folks may even be mad at me, thinking I'm stretching the truth about their favorite carbonated beverage. Each can of Coke has that same famous Nutrition Label. If you read one, you'll notice that it says there are only 100 calories. What! Is Dr. Marcotte lying?

Well, here's where the rub between nutrition experts and the food companies comes in. The food companies say they've been open and honest about what's in their products, letting people make informed decisions about their grocery shopping. The nutrition experts are mad about the same thing I'm mad about, though.

Those top two lines, the ones your eye just skips over, are the key now. This can of Coke, the one I love to crack open and down in a minute or two when I'm thirsty, is actually more than one serving! That's right, Coke apparently expects me to put the can down once I've had the 8 ounces that they say make a serving, leaving the other 4 ounces for another time.  Crazy, right?

That's the point of the fight between the nutrition experts and the food companies.  It actually gets a lot worse than this example.  What's a lousy 50 hidden calories? (8 pounds a year for those keeping score at home.)

How about the king size Snickers or the ½ liter Coke?  Maybe you favor the Big Grab bag of chips from Lays?  All of these look like one serving but are labeled as if they are 3 or 4 servings!  If you're smart enough to look at the label in the first place, you'd have to be Superman to do the math on how much of that deceptive little package is a 'serving' according to the food company and actually stop eating once you've had what they call a serving.

Even healthy seeming foods are labeled this way.  Just tonight my wife and I shared a big bag of rice cakes while I was making stir fry.  Come on, rice cakes?  What do you think I did?  Yup, turned that bag over and got progressively more ticked off as I read.

First, 70 calories catches my eye.  That's not so bad.  Then I go back above the line they want me to ignore and see 15g per serving and 12 servings per bag.  15 grams?  That's ½ ounce of rice cake.  This apparently healthy food that is not at all filling (I just ate half a bag and was still starved for supper) has just as many calories per ounce and calories per bag as any good ole fried potato chip or Dorito on the store shelves.  My wife made a conscious decision to choose the healthy food and I trusted her choice because it made sense, but we still ended up with way more calories than either of us wanted or needed in a keep-me-from-starving-before-dinner snack.

Then I looked at the garble of science terms that pass for ingredients in these rice cakes and found MSG.  That made me actually angry, so I stopped eating and went back to writing just to vent a little.

See, MSG (monosodium glutamate) is a food additive that artificially makes things taste better -- I should have known rice cakes aren't supposed to taste good. I've had to learn to watch out for this chemical since MSG always triggers a migraine for me.  I now expect to have a doozy tomorrow, just because Quaker Oats Cheddar Cheese Rice Cakes looked like a healthy snack.  I'm not the only one this affects either. There are over 20 million people with migraines in this country and many of them are sensitive to MSG.

That is truly cheating at food when you put a toxic chemical in to make folks think it tastes good.  When I find food that is made this way, it is a big strike against that company for me.

They already used half a shelf of chemicals to make "cheddar cheese flavoring" then found it still tasted bad and had to add MSG? Terrible.

If I haven't gotten you too distracted by being mad about MSG, let's go back to the piece about serving size. Some companies have just now started putting more honest labels on their food since so many doctors and nutritionists are fighting mad about it. Coke actually gets (a little) credit here because some of their cans now say '140 calories' and 'one serving' though I'm not sure how the math changed from 150 calories on the old packaging. I haven't seen the bigger bottles change the same way and until every company changes every product, I will still say we are being lied to!

The key word "serving" goes right back to the First Truth that calories count. The serving size and servings per package is incredibly important for us as we look for the truth about the foods we buy and eat. Every packaged food has this information on it and nearly every company seems to be trying to mislead us with this information. Don't believe me yet?

Spend some quality time at your local supermarket reading this labeling. Remember, the front is fair game for advertising according to the government rules, so don't even bother with the front of the package.  Pick up your favorite snack food or frozen pizza or hot dog package and turn it over.

My eyes are drawn to the **Calories**, the **Total Fat**, **Cholesterol**, **Sodium, Potassium, Total Carbohydrate**, and **Protein**.  Yours too, huh?  That's what bold print can do for information -- make some stand out and make other parts seem less important and get skipped over.  The first habit to learn is simply to turn the package over and read this boring, black-and-white panel.

As you begin this new habit, I want you to do it every time.  That's right, every packaged food or drink item needs to be read.  We need to fully realize the calories we are choosing to put in our cart and eventually into our mouths.  Remember the quote earlier?  "The truth will set you free."

In the next few pages, I want us to look at actual product labels.  Learning how to find the important parts and not be tricked by the packaging can be a little hard but is absolutely required.  With each label I have some comments and pointers, but I want you to be able to get comfortable with the details.  If you can learn how to read this stuff, you'll be prepared to choose, buy, and eat the food that will lead to a healthier you.

# Nutrition Facts

These are the 2 most important details on the label: Serving Size and Calories (per serving)

Some labels are too complicated...

These are the big 3 and always worth paying attention to

Every label has different vitamins to brag on - you can ignore this.

Serving Size  13 crackers (30g)

Servings Per Container about 6

**Amount Per Serving**

**Calories** 140    Calories from Fat  45

% Daily Value*

| | |
|---|---|
| **Total Fat** 5g | 8% |
| Saturated Fat  0.5g | 3% |
| Polunsaturated Fat  2.5g | |
| Monounsaturated Fat  1.5g | |
| Trans Fat  0g | |
| **Cholesterol** 0mg | 0% |
| **Sodium** 180mg | 8% |
| **Potassium** 170mg | 5% |
| **Total Carbohydrate** 21g | 7% |
| Dietary Fiber  3g | 12% |
| Sugars  0g | |
| **Protein** 3g | |

| | |
|---|---|
| Vitamin A  0% | Vitamin C 0% |
| Calcium  4% | Iron 6% |

*Percent Daily Values are based on a 2,000 calorie diet.

84

# Nutrition Facts

Serving Size  3 cookies (32g/1.1 oz)
Servings Per Container 1.3

**Amount Per Serving**

**Calories** 130  Calories from Fat 50

| | % Daily Value* |
|---|---|
| **Total Fat** 5g | 8% |
| Saturated Fat 2g | 10% |
| Trans Fat 0g | |
| **Cholesterol** 0mg | 0% |
| **Sodium** 170mg | 7% |
| **Total Carbohydrate** 20g | 7% |
| Dietary Fiber 2g | 6% |
| Sugars 12g | 7% |
| **Protein** 2g | |

*Percent Daily Values are based on a 2,000 calorie diet.

Look at this serving size. If you do the math, there are 4 cookies in this little pack with info on only 3! Trickery!

This little star is really important! You should know what its telling you by now. The percentages only work if you should be eating **2,000** calories per day!

Do you see the 2 columns? Most box mixes do it this way just to confuse us. Who eats the mix??

You'll see the different kinds of fats listed change - only the bold words are required, the rest is up to the company to include or not.

Who would care about getting 2% of a vitamin? This is just meant to confuse us.

The only important info below the 2nd dark line is right ⟹ here, so small you can barely read it.

# Nutrition Facts

Serving Size  1/20 pkg (26g mix)
Servings Per Container 20

| Amount Per Serving | Mix | Prepared |
|---|---|---|
| **Calories** | 100 | 170 |
| Calories from Fat | 5 | 80 |

| | % Daily Value* | |
|---|---|---|
| **Total Fat**  0.5g* | 1% | 13% |
| Saturated Fat  0g | 0% | 7% |
| Trans Fat  0g | | |
| **Cholesterol**  0mg | 0% | 7% |
| **Sodium**  90mg | 4% | 4% |
| **Potassium** 55mg | 2% | 2% |
| **Total Carbohydrate**  23g | 8% | 8% |
| Dietary Fiber  <1g | 3% | 3% |
| Sugars  15g | | |
| **Protein**  <1g | | |

| | | |
|---|---|---|
| Iron | 4% | 4% |
| Thiamin | 2% | 2% |
| Riboflavin | 0% | 2% |
| Niacin | 2% | 2% |
| Folic Acid | 2% | 2% |

*Percent Daily Values are based on a 2,000 calorie diet.

*Amount in mix. As prepared, one serving provides 9g total fat (1.5g sat. fat), 20mg cholesterol, 95mg sodium, 65mg potassium, 23g total carbohydrate (16g sugars) and 2g protein.

86

# Nutrition Facts

Serving Size  1 cup (240mL)

Servings Per Container about 2

**Amount Per Serving**

**Calories** 120   Calories from Fat 20

| | % Daily Value* |
|---|---|
| **Total Fat** 2g | 3% |
| Saturated Fat  0.5g | 3% |
| Trans Fat  0g | |
| Polyunsaturated Fat 0.5g | |
| Monounsaturated Fat 1g | |
| **Cholesterol** 15mg | 0% |
| **Sodium** 410mg | 17% |
| **Potassium** 1000mg | 29% |
| **Total Carbohydrate** 19g | 6% |
| Dietary Fiber  1g | 4% |
| Sugars  2g | 7% |
| **Protein** 7g | |

| | |
|---|---|
| Vitamin A 20% | Vitamin C 2% |
| Calcium 2% | Iron 2% |

*Percent Daily Values are based on a 2,000 calorie diet.

More funny math here. This can of soup actually has **18.6** oz. If my wife and I split the can, we both get 16 % more soup than the label admits. We all know what happens to those extra 20 calories...

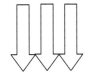

Many labels have an extra little chart down here that tells how much of each type of fat, protein, etc. we should eat based on a 2,000 calorie diet - and a 2,500 calorie diet! Not many people need 2,500 calories but up-sizing their customers is the plan...

Knowing your food is <u>required</u>. You cannot change without knowledge and you cannot learn the new eating and living habits we've been talking about without learning the truth. Experts say that learning is easiest with repetition, so I really want you to read <u>every</u> package you pick up.

Some of us will be shocked by what we see and may even now begin to change old habits and choices. "These chips have how many calories? Let's see... if I share this bag with my buddy while we watch football tomorrow that will be... 800 calories, which will take... 4 hours at the gym! Sheesh! Where are the apples?"

I'd love it if all my patients were as easy to convince as this guy. What we just imagined happening is exactly what I think needs to happen with every food choice at the beginning of our re-education about food.

Depending on whether what you've picked up is "ready-to-eat" or requires some extra steps to prepare, you may find even more information. The Apple Crisp from my pantry has 2 columns, one **Mix** and the other **As Prepared with Butter**. This makes twice as many numbers and is pretty intimidating. Well, my theory is that most food companies don't really want us to look at and understand all this stuff, so we shouldn't be surprised if it's not exactly user-friendly.

All right, back to the label.  This one says **Calories 100** (Mix column) and **200** (As Prepared with Butter column.)  There, simple right?  It only takes 20-30 minutes on the treadmill to work off if I eat the powder straight out of the box, or 40-60 minutes if I bother with mixing and baking it.  That's not so bad.  I'll bet it's a pretty nice pan of apple crisp goodness that should last me through half time of the game at least.

There is one other detail to look at though.  Remember the words above the bold line, the ones that kind of slide past your eye as you scramble to check the Calories?  Oh yeah.  I squint a little here and see "Serving Size 1/9 package" and "Servings Per Container 9"

What?  You mean my treadmill math isn't right?  Now, I've had this apple crisp.  Let me tell you, it's pretty good.  And truthfully, compared to some other desserts I could choose, one made mostly of apples is a smart nutrition choice.  The problem is that it tastes really good and seems like it's good for me, being full of apples.  That means that I can eat half the pan if I'm not paying attention.

Now what is my treadmill math with half the pan?  Since I squinted and made out the "Servings Per Container" I know that half the pan is actually 4 ½ servings... wait, 4 ½ times 200 (remember Calories As Prepared with Butter) is 900!  I should have stuck with the ½ bag of chips.

Do you get an idea of how important this is?  Can you see why I think we're being lied to?  Who knew that a seemingly healthy pan of apples (and butter, sugar, high fructose corn syrup, rolled oats, etc.) could have so many calories?

Every packaged food we choose has this same Nutrition Facts on the label.  Unfortunately, it seems like most of those foods have a random serving size that has nothing to do with how most people eat or even how the food is packaged.  Remember the 8 ounce Coke serving?  Who leaves four ounces bubbling at the bottom of the can for tomorrow?  This same thing goes on with King Size candy bars, Big Grab chips, Little Debbie snack cakes, and nearly every other snack food you can get your hands on.  Even if someone bothers to read the package, they are likely to get lulled into thinking that there are way fewer calories in the whole package than there are and, poof!  Here comes some more weight.

"Well, of course snack foods can be bad for you," you're saying.  "Everybody knows what they buy at the checkout line or the gas station is a splurge."

I wish everybody knew that - hopefully you do now. Thinking this way can get us into trouble for a couple reasons, though.  This little extra splurge is exactly the sort of thing no one remembers when they say "But I don't eat that much," and is responsible for much of the extra weight people carry around.  A Danish and latte?  That'll be 800 calories, please.  Big Gulp Coke and Big Grab Fritos? 950 calories, would you like that on your hips or thighs?

Maybe cashiers could start giving our totals like this.  That might help us make better decisions when we really want that snack.

# Caloric density

Another part of the First Truth, calories count, is that foods have dramatically different numbers of calories depending on their ingredients. Part of your higher food IQ that you're earning is that you'll be able to accurately estimate the calories in the foods you buy, prepare, order, and eat. If you have a good understanding of what goes into your body and what your body will do with it, I think you'll have made the first several steps toward a healthy diet, a healthy weight and a healthier you.

By now we've looked at Nutrition Labels enough to know several things. First, the package size and serving size may have no relationship to each other. This means that the calories that printed in the Nutrition Facts can be very misleading. As smarter food consumers, now we know how to see through that trick.

Second, food that you have to prepare may have a very different calorie count once you've added all the ingredients the instructions call for. This we can figure out too if you know how to understand and use that information.

What I want us to notice next is something that nutritionists call **Caloric Density**. Now, this won't be on the package in any easy to understand way. This is one of the things that I think food companies and restaurants are most scared that we might understand, so they won't make this easy on us.

To understand this right, we need to go back to my medical school class, Physiology. One of the most basic pieces of information we learned about food and digestion is this Caloric Density. Of course, we learned it with a bunch of scientific names and as part of a big diagram about how the body is fueled. What I want us to take from this stuffy old lecture is a few simple numbers:

Carbohydrates = 4 calories per gram

Protein = 4 calories per gram

Fat = 9 calories per gram

Alcohol = 7 calories per gram

For those of us that get a rash when we have to think about the metric system, we can translate:

Carbohydrates = 100 calories per ounce

Protein = 100 calories per ounce

Fat = 250 calories per ounce

Alcohol = 200 calories per ounce

This is where the calories that I keep harping on come from. Every food and drink can (and should!) be known by its numbers. These 3 basic building blocks (4 counting Alcohol) are what our bodies break everything we eat into. Whether we eat celery or Big Macs or filet mignon or a Mai Tai, by the end of the digestion cycle, everything that our body can use for energy (or store around our waist) gets broken down to these 4 building blocks.

What does all this have to do with Caloric Density? Good question. These numbers represent how much energy each bit of food will give our bodies. If you like numbers, you can compare Carbohydrates to Protein to Fat and see which has the most energy per gram (Fat) but what I want us to do with these numbers is kind of use them as a background to help understand the really important stuff: Caloric Density.

This is really where the rubber meets the road or where my appetite meets my waist line. What Caloric Density really means is how much do I have to sweat to burn off one mouthful of … (insert favorite food here)? Once you grasp this idea and get comfortable judging the Caloric Density of your food, you will have successfully beaten the food and restaurant companies at their own game. Ready?

Caloric Density is what makes one food choice good for your waist line and another food choice seem to go directly to your hips. Caloric Density is also the easiest and cheapest way to make things taste better, so you can bet the food companies use this to trip us up at every turn. Now, it's not really fair to compare the Caloric Density of asparagus and New York Strip or Crystal Light and Vitamin D milk. Hopefully, most of us can pick the lower calorie choice of these easy examples. But how about cream cheese and butter? Snickers and 3 Musketeers? Pretzels and potato chips? Peanut butter and jelly?

These get way more complicated but are so important if we want to learn our way through the maze of the grocery store or a restaurant menu. I want you to learn a few different ways we can judge our food and hopefully give you something you are comfortable using to make your own food choices.

Here are some rules of thumb.

1) There are more calories per mouthful (Caloric Density put another way) in anything from an animal than from a vegetable – you won't meet a fat vegetarian, and this is why!

2) Foods that are heavy for their size are usually much higher in calories – this little tip can help you decide

between the Snickers or 3 Musketeers, though I'd rather you learned to pick up an apple.

3) Adding butter, oil, dips, dressings, or cream to anything will increase its Caloric Density – remember my Apple Crisp? All those calories didn't come from the apples, I promise.

4) The softer a food is, the more likely it is to be high in calories – this has to do with how much fat or sugar is in the food. Fatty meat is tenderer than lean meat, sugary fruits are softer than healthier fruits, and more butter makes baked goods fluffier.

5) The whiter a food is, the more calories per mouthful – processing makes foods softer, whiter, smoother, and have WAY more Caloric Density. Food companies strip the coarse, healthy parts out of our food to make it prettier and more attractive but this also makes it have way more calories per mouthful.

Once you know and use these 5 rules, making good food decisions should become much simpler.

# Food Thermostat

I want to go back to an idea I mentioned earlier, the food thermostat.  To understand this idea, we need to be familiar with a real thermostat and how it works.  As a boy, I took apart almost anything I could get my hands on (to my father's chagrin) including the thermostat that kept my grandparents warm in their old house.  I remember seeing how simple it looked beneath the big plastic housing that mysteriously guarded the temperature of the living room.

Maybe you never pulled apart the family thermostat to look inside, so let me tell you what I found.  This will give us a mental picture when we start talking more about our body's food thermostat.

Inside the furnace thermostat is a lever that slides over a temperature scale, a coil of metal, and a switch.  That's it.  I know, I was surprised too when that magic thing on the wall was really so simple I could put it back together again without getting into trouble.

The furnace thermostat works because of that little metal coil which flexes based on the temperature and flips the switch, telling the furnace to turn on.  Very simple and ingenious and almost indestructible – I've pulled thermostats apart that look 100 years old and are still doing their job.  If the room temperature gets too low, the metal coil flexes enough to turn the switch on, and then once the furnace warms the room enough to reach the pre-set temperature, the coil straightens slightly and the switch turns the furnace off. Pretty cool engineering and almost foolproof. Most of these thermostats can keep a room within 2 degrees or so of the temperature we want just by a little flexible piece of metal responding to the atmosphere.

Our food thermostat is mind-bogglingly complicated but meant to do the same thing with our appetites that the wall thermostat does with the furnace. If my body gets too low on energy, the switch turns on, telling me to eat, and when I've had enough food, the switch turns off, telling me to put down my fork and wipe my mouth.

That is how our food thermostats were meant to work, anyway. If they did their job as accurately as the wall thermostats in our houses do theirs, I could save a lot of ink and paper and not bother with this book.

The truth is that for many reasons our food thermostats are nowhere near as precise as a wall thermostat even in the best of situations. Worse, some people's thermostats don't seem to work at all anymore. As I said earlier, our food thermostats were life-and-death important when our ancestors were cavemen or pioneers.

We are born with an accurate thermostat that is good at waking Mom and Dad up every couple of hours to nurse or fix the bottle. Almost every baby's thermostat works normally in the first few months of life, turning on the tears and screams when the body gets hungry and then turning off the tears and going to sleep when the hunger is satisfied.

So what happened to that efficient and accurate thermostat we were born with? Why is it so far off for most adults?

There are many reasons our thermostats can be off, maybe as many reasons as there are people, but I think most of the reasons fall into a few categories. If we can understand the reasons our thermostats are out of whack and misleading, then we can learn to interpret them accurately and even heal them.

As I said, babies are born with very precise food thermostats. Most toddlers have highly accurate food thermostats as well. So when and why did most of us get off track?

I think habit is the single biggest reason our food thermostats get warped. Sadly, these habits are usually started when we are kids, as young as two or three. Something outside of our body started trying to control when and how much we ate, often for what seemed like good reasons at the time.

"Clean your plate."

"If you don't try at least a bite, you can't have any dessert."

"Snack time."

Humans are very good at adapting, learning, and changing. If you learned that the foods you wanted might be hard to get again later, you might have adapted by eating more than your food thermostat told you to, trying to make sure you got your share. Being made to clean your plate before you could leave the table or being made to stay at the table past the point of being done eating could easily teach you to keep eating beyond what your food thermostat was telling you to eat.

School snacks or afternoon snacks with your friends in mom's kitchen might have been your first exposure to social eating. The pressure to eat what everyone else was eating, even if you weren't hungry or didn't particularly like what was being served could easily warp your sense of being hungry or full.

Once our food thermostats stop being reliable, we start to depend on another way to tell when to be done eating. For one person, that's when the plate is clean, for another that's when everyone is done eating. Another person might not be done until dessert is finished and all the leftovers are put away.  Whatever the signal to our mouths to stop chewing, it's not as good as the one we were born with.

The bad thing about this new signal to stop eating is that it has just as much power as the original one without the fine-tuned control.  Now I stay hungry and keep eating until everyone at the table is finished with their dinner.  If you ask me why I'm still eating, I can honestly say it's because I'm still hungry -- my eyes are now the boss of my appetite, not my stomach or metabolism.

As you can guess, this change in the food thermostat can causes big problems for people and is usually one of the hardest parts of a person's life to change if they want to permanently change their weight.  The good news is that the food thermostat **can** be restarted and **can** learn to work correctly again.  The bad news is that it isn't quick or easy to make this happen.

Restarting the food thermostat requires a person to ignore the signals their body uses for hunger until that habit or collection of habits is broken.  Here's where the hard part of a diet comes in, the feeling of hunger and self-deprivation, because the broken food thermostat must be ignored until it shuts off.  If it weren't broken folks wouldn't have the weight problems they do.

Re-training a food thermostat is slow but absolutely necessary. The feeling of being hungry all the time while on a 'diet' is the main reason people can't stick to their diets and will usually give up. Then of course they often regain whatever weight they lost plus a little bonus. That hunger is not true. It is a false feeling, but it sure is a powerful one.

Here is one of the reasons I am such a big fan of group programs like Weight Watchers. As I've said, millions of people have the same fight with their bodies. Why do it alone? Knowing that others are fighting too can be a big boost and can even give you practical tips on how others have fought and won.

A person's food thermostat can absolutely be reset, tuned to truly tell when they are hungry instead of when some other signal comes in to tell them to eat. If you get hungry when you sit down at the table and don't feel full until everyone is ready to get up, you can have your thermostat re-trained. If your appetite starts up whenever you get stressed or bored, it doesn't have to be that way. If an empty plate is the only way you know how to feel full, that can change.

What absolutely must come first, though, is the desire to change, the want to. From the beginning I've told you I can't make you do anything or even make you want to do anything. The same goes here.

One of the most essential ways to start re-training your food thermostat is to know exactly what, when, and how much you eat. The two-week food diary I suggested earlier is very important here. A person must have knowledge before they can change. Tracking your food, drink, and water for a two-week period is a great way to start learning about your body and your appetite.

Once your two-week food diary is done, you should probably make an appointment with your family doctor and get some help finding the calorie traps in your diet. If your family doctor isn't comfortable helping you like this (and some won't be) just ask for a referral to a dietician at the local hospital. These folks are the true experts and can help you a lot. Any way you do it, track your calories and find out where your traps are.

The next step in re-training your food thermostat is to calculate how many calories your body needs for a day. Lots of websites can help you calculate this if you hate math, but the equations I gave on page 50 are a good place to start. Your daily calorie need is the starting point for re-learning how to eat and when to stop eating.

You will need to plan your diet out in detail for the next two weeks. Now is when you start really using the information you learned from your food diary and your doctor or dietician plus the number of calories your body needs each day. Again, the Internet can be a useful source of information (as long as you are careful whose advice you listen to) and there are good diabetes education sites that can help you plan a detailed menu for two weeks or longer based on how many calories you and your doctor have calculated you should have.

Once you get this diet made, it's time to jump in and do it. Oh yeah, and your hunger signals for this two weeks? They must be ignored as part of re-training your food thermostat. If you make a balanced diet that is enough calories based on our calculations, you <u>will not</u> starve and any hunger symptoms you have are FALSE and must be ignored.

The good news is that your body and mind will begin to adapt during those two weeks and it won't be as hard at the end as it is going to be at the beginning. The bad news is that it will be hard at the beginning and you'll be tempted to quit. Don't! This is worth it and you've got to push through the hard part if you want to ever win your fight with your weight.

# Artificial Sweeteners

All our talk of food and calories leads us next to talk about some of the fakes people have come up with over the years. Loving sweet things to eat is a basic human fact. Probably about the same time our food thermostat developed our ancestors started liking and then looking for sweets.

Thousands of years ago, summer fruits and the occasional honeybee hive were the only sweet things to be found. Both of these were good to add to a boring and often bad diet of meat and grains. The sweets were so rare and life was so hard that growing fat from fruit or honey wasn't very likely.

In more recent times, people learned to keep bees for easier access to honey and then to grow sugar cane or sugar beets to harvest sugar itself, making sweet foods far more common. Our basic human love of sweets is still going strong, but now instead of a rare treat to add to a hunter's diet, sugar or sweetener is added to nearly every processed food we buy.

We talked earlier about our appetites not being able to tell when we got calories from our drinks. Sugar and sweeteners are the main place these calories come from. As you can guess, I'm not the first person to figure out that drinking sweet pop or tea all day can make a person fat. In fact, a whole industry of artificial sweeteners has been growing for many years. The oldest commonly known artificial sweetener is saccharin, discovered in the late 1800's by chemists in Europe (there is some argument about who gets credit and when exactly it happened.) Even a hundred years ago it was known that saccharin was sweet but not sugar and gave no extra calories to food or drink.

Since then, the search for more sugar-like chemicals without sugar-like calories has made plenty of people rich but not many skinny. Why not? It seems like this is the perfect solution to our sugar cravings fighting against our waists. It is so obvious that scientists have even found a substitute for fat, our other universal craving. That chemical, olestra, has its own interesting side effects that would make a good story too.

Here, I want to focus on the artificial sweeteners not because of side effects (though they certainly exist) or taste (because not many people are fooled into thinking they are actually sugar) but because of another effect they seem to have.

Though there is argument among scientists, it looks as if the most common artificial sweetener, aspartame (NutraSweet, Equal) can actually increase appetite. This is a very complicated topic, probably because there is so much money involved, but many people seem to be hungrier and eat more if they have this artificial sweetener with or before a meal.

Isn't that crazy?  We already learned that sugary drinks are ignored by the appetite, just adding calories to our fast food lunches.  Now it looks as if the diet drinks that seem like a better choice may make us eat even more!  Do you see where I get my conspiracy theory from?  It sure feels like somebody wants us all to be fatter.

So what to do?  First I bash juice, saying you might as well have a Coke and vitamin pill rather than drinking everybody's favorite, orange juice.  Then I jump straight in and start hollering about how bad soda pop is for us and how I think juice and pop are a big reason Americans are so big.  Now, of all things, I'm telling you that even diet pop may be part of the problem.  AHHHHH!!!

Is that how some of you are feeling?  I'm sorry, I wish it wasn't so, but all these things are true and all of them affect every one of us.  As you can guess, I don't think the solution comes from better chemistry.

The solution, the only solution is to change what, when, how and why we eat.  I'll say it again: **no one can eat like an American and not get fat**.  We are the fattest country on earth but countries that are catching up to us are catching up <u>because they are starting to eat like us</u>.  Once

McDonald's seems like a normal part of life, once typical American restaurant food (huge servings with lots of hidden calories) becomes something other than a rare part of a person's diet, here comes the weight.

I hope you can hear this and really begin to take it in. We really do have to change our way of living and our way of eating if we want to lose weight, feel better, and live healthier. Now, don't get me wrong, I like a juicy steak or a bowl of ice cream as much as the next person. And I think by now you know I enjoy a cold Coke even more than a lot of folks do.

I'm not telling you, me, or anyone to stop eating things we like. I am telling all of us that we must change **how much** and **how often** we eat those things. Some of them are so bad for me that I may only enjoy them once a month or less. The nurses in my office will nudge each other and point when they see me with a Coke. They know how often I lecture about it but also how rarely I have one.

This is the kind of change that I'm describing. Nothing is completely off the list of eating possibilities. A lot of things need to come off our regular shopping and dining out lists, though. We really have no choice if we want to lose weight and feel better. Tradeoffs must be made; our calorie needs

<u>must</u> be obeyed.  The only other option is a life-long struggle with weight and bad health.

If the math says you can have 2,000 calories a day without gaining weight, I hope you know by now that 2,001 calories a day every day will add up and 2,500 calories a day will add up fast.

There is truly no way around that, no miracle drug or diet or activity that can make you the exception.  No matter how often you hear a company or a person promise they have a loophole, fight the urge to believe it – it's not true!

# Exercise is Good for You – But...

Every day I risk confusing my patients.  Most of my long-term patients can tell you that I usually ask about how they are eating and if they are exercising.  Since these two things are already linked in most people's mind I just add to it by asking it this way.  Truth be told, it's an old habit for me, a way of making sure I get all the important questions into a patient's visit.  Now and then somebody brings this up in our conversation and reminds me that I've been misleading my patients again.

The truth is that eating 'right' and getting exercise are both very important and often are present (or absent) in people's life together, but aren't linked the way folks think they are.  Most people put eating right and getting some exercise in the same "I-ought-to-be-doing-but-don't" sentence.  This connection has probably come from us doctors because the combination is very important for heart health and diabetes treatment and cholesterol control and lots of other chronic illnesses.

Maybe because healthy eating and exercising are often mentioned together in the doctor's office, they seem to be stuck together in people's mind.  I even hear people tell me they won't even try to do one unless they dedicate themselves to both.  Either habit is hard to make by itself, but if you think that both have to run together then it can seem like an impossible goal and not even worth trying.

That sense of "No way could I do that" is common in my patients. Whenever I hear this sort of discouragement I try to separate the two goals and give people permission to pick one to try out, saving the other to worry about for later. Either regular exercise or an improved diet is very good for you and I am always thrilled to find a patient who has successfully started either change in their life.

Judging by how excited I get when someone starts either habit and by how often I ask about each habit, it's easy to see how they get linked in people's minds. So I get reminded of this connection most of the time when I have an angry patient, upset that I have 'misled' them and wanting me to fix it. *Misleading my patients? How terrible! I would never... Oh yeah, they think that exercising will make them lose weight. Dang it.* That's my inner voice every time this comes up and that's why this is part of my book.

Do you remember earlier, chapters ago when I talked about my gym manager being mad at me? I want to go back to that again and remind us all of the Second Truth. **You can't exercise your way to weight loss.** My angry patients are finding this truth out for themselves and often feel like I've misled them into thinking that they can lose weight with exercise.

Once the topic comes up, we talk about it at length, me giving them the can of Coke illustration (two minutes to drink, thirty minutes to burn off) and eventually we are friends again. What I don't want, what I almost beg them, is to not quit exercising.

A habit of walking or jogging or biking or swimming can add years to your life, prevent common diseases, give you more energy, improve your mood, and even improve your metabolism by building muscle. These are great things, stuff that pills and doctors just can't give you, things I want for my patients and they want for themselves.

So if you already have a good exercise habit, please don't give it up. Nothing could be better for you. Just don't count on it making you slim. Only professional athletes and people that put in that much effort can expect to lose weight by exercise alone. Thirty minutes a day on the treadmill or bike is great for you and your heart but won't change your waist very much. Why? Say it with me: "Calories matter." That's right, back to the same old saying – because it's true.

Think of it this way: Would you expect combing your hair to prevent cavities? Would buckling your seatbelt be very likely to get you a raise? Some actions have expected results and exercise is one of them. You should expect exercise to make you feel better, often in several ways. Your stamina and breathing will probably get better, your muscle tone will probably get better, and your mood and stress level will probably get better. Your weight? Maybe, but don't count on it. Remember, 3,500 calories make a pound and 30 minutes of walking burns 150 calories. That makes 12 hours of fast walking to burn off one pound. Ugh. The math on exercising for weight loss isn't pretty. The other benefits exercise can give you? Wonderful.

Pick an activity you don't hate, find a place to do it no matter what the weather, carve out the hour in your busy day, and get to it. Unfortunately, like my food advice, it's simple but far from easy. Here the reward is different than what I've promised if you'll change your diet.

Eat fewer calories, lose weight. That's been my only promise so far (besides promising that if you ignore this advice, your waist will show it!) Here I'll make another promise: exercise regularly and feel better.

That's it? That's it. Your body is willing to bribe you. If you want to feel better or lose weight, there are only a couple of bribes that will work over the long haul. Lots of late-night infomercials and ladies magazine glossy ads will tell you another story but guess what, they're trying to sell you something. The lies go where the money is, remember? I'm

116

not trying to sell you anything (except my book) so I don't have any reason to lie to you.

This is all true. The bribes that will work between you and your body are very simple.

**Exercise, feel better.**

**Eat fewer calories, lose weight.**

Keep going back to those two sentences, read them as often as it takes to really sink in. Helping you believe and decide to live by these simple decisions is why I wrote all this. Don't brush this off or put off deciding for later. How you feel and feel about yourself <u>for the rest of your life</u> comes down to simple decisions like these. How often you need to see your doctor could very well come down to simple decisions like these too.

Exercise really does make you feel better. Lots of research has proven this but getting your own real-life testimony may be more important than a bunch of scientists spouting off about *endorphins* and *oxygen carrying capacity*. So go ask around. You'll find folks willing to tell you about how good going to the gym or running, biking, swimming, whatever makes them feel. This isn't baloney or people lying to themselves or even people wired differently than you. It's simply true.

You can find plenty of people who can come up with good reasons not to exercise (maybe you're one of them?) You can find lots of folks who are dedicated to their sport or workout. Not as many people have (accidently) done an experiment on themselves and are able to tell you from the inside how different exercising or couch potato-ing can make you feel.

I have done this accidental experiment on myself at least twice now over the last 20 years. I have gone from dedicated exerciser to maker of excuses and back again twice. I now know very well how much better I feel in every way when I get back into regular exercise. My mood improves (ask my wife), my energy climbs, I'm more immune to all the germs people bring into my office, I even get more efficient with my time so I don't miss the hour I carve out for the gym.

I'm telling you, this works. It has for me and millions of other people and it can work for you too. Better mood, energy and stamina can't be bought but they can be earned. It's worth it!

# So What Should I Eat?

Maybe some of you are getting frustrated with me, always telling you what <u>not</u> to do, what <u>not</u> to eat. Some folks learn better by focusing on the positives and wish I'd get a little more positive.

A while back we talked about the linebacker and the couch potato, remember? Most of what we talked about way back then before you learned all this stuff about calories and waistlines was focused on proving that everyone has the same metabolism. I did mention a little about lean meat for the linebacker but didn't get into it much.

Now I think we're ready to dig into what to eat though we'll always keep the calorie count in mind as we figure this part out. You could probably fill a small library with the books people have written about what to eat and what not to, but as you've seen I like things simple and I want to keep this part simple too.

Some books say to eat all protein, others say to eat all carbohydrates and some talk about stranger things like the cookie diet or the soup diet. Subway Jared has a career based on his sandwich diet and there is a taco place advertising the drive-thru diet.

Some folks swear we were meant to be vegetarian, others joke about being a "meat-etarian" and people think Dr. Adkins told everyone to eat only bacon and lard. The government has spent lots of time and money coming up with their Pyramids telling us how much of what to eat and dairy farmers are spending lots of money telling us to drink 3 glasses of milk a day to lose weight.

When you add all the diet pills, herbs, and supplements that folks sell and swear by, the possibilities are endless. Unfortunately, the profits are huge and the results are tiny from all these choices.

By now hopefully you can guess what I say about all these diets – say it with me: **Calories Count**. Any of these diets can probably work if they can trick people into cutting their calories. Most of the effort and planning is spent on trying to trick people's brains and appetites into thinking they are eating 'whatever you want' but still losing weight. The truth is 'whatever you want' is probably true but 'as much as you want' will have to wait on that magic pill we all wish for.

So if I'm not going to tell you to eat all cookies or all bacon or no fat or only cabbage soup, what is my advice? All the complicated scientific stuff you might hear from a good Dietician or Nutritionist can be boiled down to this:

> **Be a food racist – Don't Eat White.**

That's it?  Yup, that's it.

This really can get as complicated as you want to make it but I like things simple and easy to understand and remember. If you asked my patients what they remember me telling them, hopefully the first thing would be something about smoking.  I'll bet right after that would be this quote.  I settled on this several years ago as the simplest, best way to stick what I wanted my patients to do into their heads.

That's what I want to do for you too.  Become a food racist – Don't Eat White.  "OK," you say, "I'll try to keep it in my head – but what does it mean?"  Are you sure it's in there now?  I meant it; I really want this to stick.  So, one more time: Be a food racist – Don't Eat White.

Now that my crazy little saying is swimming around in your head, let's figure out what it means.  The 'racist' part is just meant to get your attention and hopefully won't offend anyone of any race – this is talking about food, folks.  What I said about white I meant, though – Don't Eat White.

Why the hang-up on food color?  What have I got against white?  I think this is the easiest way to pick out the foods that have had all the nutrition taken out, the foods that have been processed to the point that the calories are empty or at least less good for you than they could be.  Remember,

121

the calories still count, they <u>always</u> count, so picking foods that give us something more than calories is definitely better, kind of a bonus.

The other reason this matters goes back to our Fourth Truth. You remember? You are becoming what you eat. The white food is also the soft, fluffy, filled-with-chemicals food and <u>not</u> what you want your body made from, I promise.

I have the most luck convincing people about this when they first find out they are pregnant. A lady and her husband are sitting in my office, waiting for the happy (or shocking) news. Shortly after I congratulate them and write her a prescription for prenatal vitamins, I remind her that her baby is a tiny lump of cells that will be growing like crazy for the next several months. What she eats is what her baby will be made of. I know she's heard me when I see the shock in her eyes. "Do you want your baby to be made of McDonald's or healthy food?"

Moms have told me this can really help control their cravings later in pregnancy and I think it helps control mom's weight gain too. What I really hope it does, what I push for over their child's first few months and years of life, is a change in what the whole family eats.

Yes, that baby boy will be completely made from whatever his mommy eats while she is pregnant. But he will also be made from whatever he eats the rest of his life, mom will be made from whatever she eats, and dad will be too. It's that simple. **We are all becoming what we eat**, nothing more and nothing less.

Whatever I put in my mouth is all my cells get to repair themselves and make more cells, which is all I am. The chemicals, preservatives, and additives in my food become part of me. The chemicals, preservatives, and additives in your food become part of you.

One of the funniest and most shocking movies I've seen is Super-Size Me. I recommend this to patients frequently and recommend it to you too. The director, Morgan Spurlock, has become famous for doing crazy things for 30 days and filming it, just to see what it's like. In this movie, he decides to eat only McDonald's, three meals a day, for thirty days. He has 3 doctors he sees weekly during this time, who chart his body's changes and do blood testing on him to see how bad his cholesterol gets. It is shocking and amazing to watch this fit, healthy guy who hates fast food gain over 20 pounds and make himself so sick that one of his doctors orders him to stop, all the while craving McDonald's more and more. You really should watch it.

My favorite part isn't part of the movie, though. The DVD has extras at the end and a couple have stuck in my mind for years after watching. One of the extras is about his recovery from his month of McDonald's. It takes him almost a year to lose the weight he gained in that month (see, more proof that it's much easier to never put it in your mouth in the first place.) It takes his liver months to recover from the shock he gave it. I get the idea that it took his girlfriend, a vegetarian health nut, months to forgive him too though she must have because they are married now.

The other part that I remember so well is actually a little experiment he did with the McDonald's food. He ordered a hamburger, a Big Mac, a Filet-O-Fish and a large fry and put them on his desk. He also ordered a burger and fries from a neighborhood place down the street. Then he filmed them every day for weeks to see what happened.

Maybe I shouldn't tell you – it is pretty gross. Or maybe I should leave you hanging so you'll go rent it and see for yourself. Nah, I've gotta tell you.

The food from the eatery down the street molded and then turned to nasty goop within just a few days on his desk. The McDonald's food? Weeks to even sprout mold. The Big Mac looked completely edible three weeks later. It took months for the McDonald's sandwiches, bun and all, to rot. And the worst part? The fries. They sat on his desk for <u>over 10 months</u> and still looked like they did the day he ordered them! Who knows how long they might have lasted had his film school intern not thrown them away by mistake.

Now do you see what I'm saying about food preservatives and chemicals becoming a part of you? Something that even mold and bacteria can't digest is every kid's favorite food? Ahhhhhhh!

The good news about our bodies being made of what we eat is that it's never too late to change. Maybe we've had too many burgers making our waists too big and maybe all the preservatives are swimming around in our system making us unhealthy. Maybe we feel tired and have no energy and are teetering into depression all the time. Maybe all this news about what we've been doing to our one and only body for years is getting us down. But you know what? This same body that has built itself out of whatever we've been eating will continue to rebuild itself over and over every day as long as we live.

What that means is that whenever we decide to change and turn our eating habits around, our bodies will immediately begin building with the good stuff we start giving them. **No matter how unhealthy we've been, we can always start making it better.** Almost every part of you has been remade many, many times. New cells grow and replace older ones, new molecules and atoms replace the ones that used to be there and nothing stays the same for long.

Too much McDonald's stuck here and there? Too many Snickers or Frito's or cigarettes wedged in between the Big

Macs? That's all right, your body will forgive you and start to bribe you with feeling good just as soon as you turn your eating habits around and start giving it healthy building blocks. This is a change worth making too, a change that will pay you back over and over for years to come if you'll put the time and effort into making the change.

# Changing

How do we make all these healthy changes?  As I've said all along, these changes are simple but none of them are easy. I think making a change takes 4 different ingredients: Ability to Change, Desire to Change, Knowledge of What to Change, and Motivation to Change.

The **Ability to Change** is probably the easiest of the four ingredients to talk about because it is pretty much automatic.  Any responsible adult person has proven they <u>can</u> change just by getting to the point where they can be called a 'responsible adult.'  Life is full of unexpected things that constantly require us to grow and change and adapt.  If a person truly can't change, they can't make it in the world. Someone will have to take care of them and make decisions for them. So, what do you think?  Do you pass the Ability to Change test?  I thought so.

The **Desire to Change** is a little more difficult to prove to someone, though I suspect you don't really need me to prove this to you.  Who doesn't want to change, to improve, to be better?  That too is a natural part of being human.  The fact that you picked up this book and stuck with me to this point is the best proof that you have the Desire to Change. See?  Two down and we haven't even broken a sweat.

What about **Knowledge of What to Change**? Not long ago, this was in doubt. As we've talked about, there is plenty of bad information and outright lies to be heard about food and exercise. Most of us have heard and believed many of those lies for years. Remember what you used to think about juice? White bread? Maybe even McDonald's? Hopefully I've taught you some truths that are fighting the lies. Once those truths settle into your head and become easy and automatic for you to believe, then I would say the Knowledge of What to Change is a done deal.

That just leaves one thing. Change requires Ability, Desire, Knowledge... and Motivation.

As you can guess, this is the crucial part, the part I can't give you or convince you that you already have. What will motivate you, how to motivate you, isn't something I can know. I do know that it is essential though. I know that without motivation all the rest of the ingredients are just decoration – they may look nice but they won't cause Change.

Even though knowing how to get the **Motivation to Change** is something only you and people that know and love you can know for you, I want to give you some examples to start you thinking and maybe 'motivate you to find your motivation.'

A very common motivation is *dissatisfaction*. This motivation works well for me. This is why I refer to the bribes your body is willing to offer you and talk so much about feeling good and feeling bad. If you dislike how life and your health or weight is enough, you may get Motivated to Change. Part of the problem here is knowing just how much a person has to dislike the present to reach motivation. Again, only you can know that about you and if you are already Motivated to Change by being dissatisfied, stop reading and go for it!

Other people are more motivated by the *needs of others*. Women that smoke always find quitting easiest when they are pregnant. Knowing what they do affects someone they love very much is enough motivation to make Change easy. Having a baby is often what it takes to shock a tough guy into taking his own health seriously. Having a little someone look up at you and knowing that you want to be there and healthy for them for many years to come may be exactly the Motivation to Change you need to. If so, get to it!

Other folks get their motivation juices going with a little healthy *competition*. Maybe you need to make a friendly bet with your spouse or sister or co-worker about who can reach a certain health goal the quickest.  Having someone to push and encourage you may be all you need to get going toward your goal of being healthier.  If you don't yet have someone that will join you in the competition, maybe you need to push them a little, get them interested or buy them this book (Husbands, not a good birthday or Christmas gift idea here!)  Once you get that start then go do it!

Similar to the competitive type of motivation is *accountability*.  This is what makes Weight Watchers so successful for so many people.  It is simpler and cheaper and more 'do-able' than any other program out there.  What really makes it go, though, is the weekly weigh-in.  Knowing other people will know if you've been following through on your promises to them and yourself is a very strong motivation for some people and may be for you.  If this type of Motivation to Change works for you, then make it happen!

The examples I've given so far – dissatisfaction, competition, accountability, and the needs of others – are all good Motivations to Change and most people will find that at least one works strongly for them.  Some folks may find other motivations and I say whatever works, use it.

There is one other motivation that I saved until last. It is the strongest motivator but also the worst and scariest. I really hope you never even meet this motivator, let alone wait on it to find you before you change, though many of my patients do.

This last and worst motivator is *catastrophe*. Waiting until the heart attack comes to eat right and exercise, throwing away the cigarettes after the cancer is found, skipping the drive-thru only once you get diagnosed with diabetes. That's what I mean by catastrophe being the last, strongest, worst motivator. I just hope you don't wait for that sort of a wake-up call. Please pick another Motivation to Change and use it to avoid these health catastrophes.

Now it's time to put down the book and get to it! Go be the healthy change you want for yourself – start today!!

Thanks for joining me!

Now the journey begins – join me online for more education, encouragement, and motivation:

http://DoctorFoodTruth.com

Twitter: @DoctorFoodTruth

12194981R00075

Made in the USA
Charleston, SC
19 April 2012